I0767184

To Walk In

Faith

Twenty-One Days to Walk in the Power of Faith

Sandra J. Petrusaitis

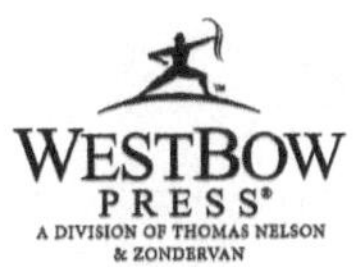

WestBow
PRESS®
A DIVISION OF THOMAS NELSON
& ZONDERVAN

WestBow Press books may be ordered through booksellers or by contacting:

WestBow Press
A Division of Thomas Nelson & Zondervan
1663 Liberty Drive
Bloomington, IN 47403
www.westbowpress.com
1 (866) 928-1240

Interior Image Credit: Mark Schwartz

ISBN: 978-1-9736-6577-9 (sc)
ISBN: 978-1-9736-6578-6 (hc)
ISBN: 978-1-9736-6576-2 (e)

Library of Congress Control Number: 2019907525

Print information available on the last page.

WestBow Press rev. date: 11/20/2019

Contents

DEDICATION

To women created as glorious and beautiful beings to reflect God's very image. In you, beloved, God planned the future of mankind in all its glory and splendor. In the holiness of His peace, He created and fashioned you to live in His glorious light, to give birth to hope, to bear the fruit of love, and to give grace its pulsing heartbeat. It's your time, beloved, to rise and walk as the woman He created, in His image, and take hold of all His promises. The kingdom of God is eagerly waiting for His beloved daughters to rise and to walk upright in God's light.

Introduction

This is a new season for us in this ministry. Working with Mark Schwartz, artist and shoe designer, has given us not only great insight about the fashion and beauty worlds but also a common thread and passion for all things beautiful. You can find more information on his art and designs, along with his many accolades and expertise, on his website, www.highheeledart.com. We are very excited and look forward to the success of this project and to many more collaborations and partnerships.

As a culture, we may see spiritual matters as things that exist on the fringes. You only need to read the headlines to see where we could be heading unless we find the common ground of grace.

We often believe that it is one side or another. I believe we have forgotten that our spiritual nature is in our DNA. Denying our spiritual nature is like denying our next breath. We may not see it, but it's in our spirit, where we can achieve the ultimate potential of peace and goodwill.

We may vary in our beliefs; however, we each desire the safety of our loved ones and peace in our communities.

Because I will never be able to deny how much I love being a woman and how much I love fashion, I chose to use shoes as the symbol of our daily walk in and through Christ. As Americans, we sometimes take for granted that we have choices.

Why shoes? Shoes remind me how easy it is to walk in certain attitudes. They also remind me how easy it can be to change your attitude. When you look at a woman fully dressed, her shoes tell the story of where she intends to go.

I've always admired shoes. My earliest memory of admiring them was an Easter Holiday. When I saw a little girl wearing a pair of white patent leather shoes with a white pom-pom at the top. The frilly pom-poms made it seem as if she was dancing with every step.

What shoes a woman chooses to wear is a tell of what roads she's willing to tread. Athletic or sporty shoes are more dynamic and suggest a "can-do, will do" attitude. Wearing high-heeled shoes is a bold statement. Reflecting what heights she's aspiring and willing to go. While boots are meant to be worn for protection. A demonstration of preparedness for what comes her way.

Sandals, while protecting the most delicate part of the feet also speak to being carefree yet ready for the journey. Just as being barefoot in the Bible refers to the intimacy of being in God's holy presence. A woman who is barefoot may be a way she shows her level of comfort or her vulnerability.

Shoes are so profoundly a simple representation of our

spiritual journey. Perhaps we need to survey our innate spiritual connection to a Holy God just as simply.

My hope is that as you read this book, you may connect with the simplicity of wearing shoes, and become more aware of your spiritual being, of the hope, the grace and the blessings of coming to intimately know God as our Heavenly Father.

Chapter 1: Woman

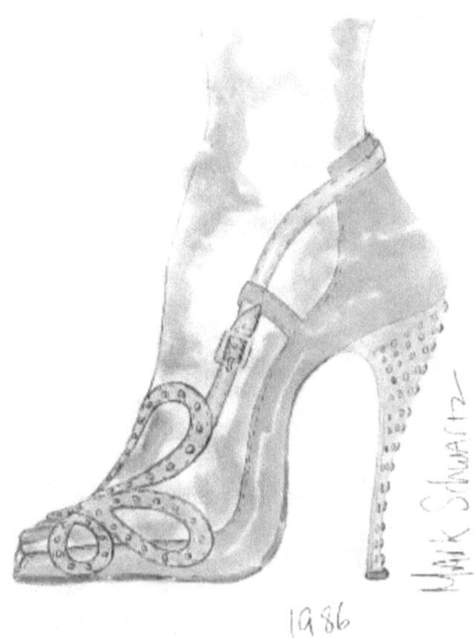

"Her Majesty Queen Elizabeth II commissioned Roger Vivier to design the shoes for her coronation day. On June 2, 1953, he was the only French designer to attend the royal crowning ceremony.

In 1986, as a design exercise, Vivier asked me to sketch an updated version of his famous coronation shoe. Above is my version: watercolor on sketch paper, from the Mark Schwartz personal archive."

What is it about woman that has so intrigued humanity ever since her creation? Woman was fashioned to be spectacular. Her impact and influence could not be contained in that one moment God intended for her in His heart. As if His love for her sent out shockwaves throughout eternity with an intensity that echoes and reverberates with every beat of her heart today. Her truth was veiled yet not quite hidden, obvious and not grasped.

Almost since her creation, woman has been vilified or magnified—a woman like you, who is unique and beautiful. She's either deprecated or elevated to the status of goddess. While on the one hand, she is a wonder, on the other, she becomes denigrated.

Throughout history, we've either been mystified by her powers or burned her for her craft. She is exploited and allows herself to be exploited all at once. She understands her feminine power to a measure, then becomes a victim of her very nature.

In the garden, God put Adam into a deep sleep before He created her (Genesis 2:21 AKJV). God forged her out of Adam's rib. The serpent then entered the garden and deceived her. Adam blamed her, and to this day, she is the reason for post-modern psychotherapy.

We love her, and we hate her. She is beautiful, and her bitterness will destroy all those who cross her path. Her wrath is historical. Her beauty has captivated nations, and her heroism has led many to freedom. Destined to give birth to the Savior of the world, she is still the subject of debate over her reputation and purity. She has suffered under the vengeful hand of the authorities and has been the central character of *The Da Vinci Code.*

We hail her for rearing socially adept children yet chastise her for not being functional and viable out of the home. We love her as the bride but hate her as the mother-in-law. She is confident with her youth and beauty yet critiqued for her lack of purity.

Yet, in Christ, she is the woman with the issue of blood, a woman forgiven for adultery and spared from death. She sits at His feet and hears His voice. Through Him, we know her to be of noble character, wise and selfless. God engenders wisdom as feminine. He speaks of her place in beauty and her holiness. In Song of Solomon, He celebrates her love, her righteousness, and her beauty. In Proverbs, He considers her more valuable than rubies.

The woman at the well is remembered for her fervor to evangelize. She is accounted as the first to take the good news of the Gospel to the people.

Although her being is never disputed, there is a very real call for woman to arise. In her, God has added not only a womb that gives life but also the power to submit all she is and will be. Christ describes her as the bride, the promise of His return. And in Revelation, she gives birth to light only to be captured into heaven.

Woman, God (Elohim) created you and formed you with

His hands in an environment of intense intimacy and peace in the garden. And as He stood before you, His breath gave you life. In peace, He created you; in love, He predestined you to be His daughter through Christ. From creation to this moment, He is with you. He never left and wants you to see yourself through His eyes. You already possess the divine characteristics and traits you exhaustively seek. He is your ever-living, gloriously omniscient, and ever-loving God (Elohim), our Father, through our sovereign Lord, Christ Jesus. From your creation to this moment, God has never left your side. You are woman, daughter, sister, mother, and friend. And in Christ, you are a child of the Resurrection—a child of the Highest God.

Chapter 2: Why Were You Created?

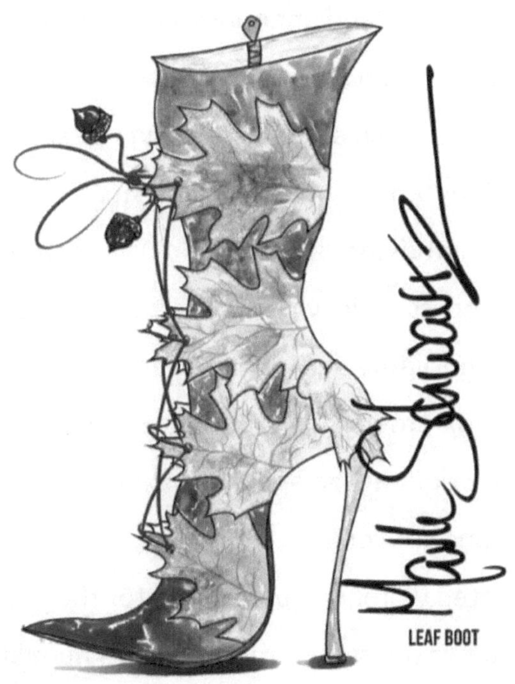

Why did God create you? Why right here and right now? The truth is that we all ask this question. The moment we can reason, we not only ask the question we also passionately pursue the answer.

God isn't offended by our questions, just as a teacher is not offended by a child asking a simple question from a child's perspective. The Bible is written as an answer to our questions. The Bible is a man-written, Holy Spirit–inspired publication. It is truly where others, no differently from us today, pursued and asked that very question. Man asked, "God, who are You? Why am I here? What's all this life thing about?" God's response to His creation is "In the beginning, God …" (Genesis 1:1 KJV).

In Luke, we read that when the archangel appeared to Zechariah in the temple and announced that Elizabeth, his wife, was to conceive a child and that his name was to be John (Luke 1:11–13 AKJV), Zechariah asked, "How *can* I be sure of this? I am an old man, and my wife is well along in years." The Bible says the angel struck him silent until the child was born. Zechariah's question answered itself, leaving God out of the answer. However, when the archangel came to Mary and announced the birth of Jesus, Mary asked, "How *will* this be, since I know not a man?" Her question put God right at the apex of the answer. Ask Him, and He will lovingly answer you.

God created woman equal to man for the purpose of being equal and greater at the same time. She is his humility. He is her strength.

So, to answer the first question, "Why did God create you?" I'd love to tell you that the answer is simple. However, it would take me much longer to elaborate and guide you to unfold the answer. This is more of a question for you to ponder, because the truth is that the answer to this question is a unique journey for two: you and your Creator.

I do encourage you to ask the questions to the one who can answer them. Pursue it, ponder it, meditate on it, fasten your seatbelt, and then enjoy the most extraordinary journey of your life!

How Much God Says He Loves You

> Behold, what manner of love the Father hath bestowed upon us, that we should be called the sons of God: therefore the world knoweth us not, because it knew him not. (1 John 3:1 KJV)

> For I am convinced that neither death nor life, neither angels nor demons, neither the present nor the future, nor any powers, neither height nor depth, nor anything else in all creation, will be able to separate us from the love of God that is in Christ Jesus our Lord. (Romans 8:38–39 NIV)

> But because of his great love for us, God, who is rich in mercy, made us alive with Christ even when we were dead in transgressions—it is by grace you have been saved. (Ephesians 2:4–5 NIV)

Chapter 3: Unconnected

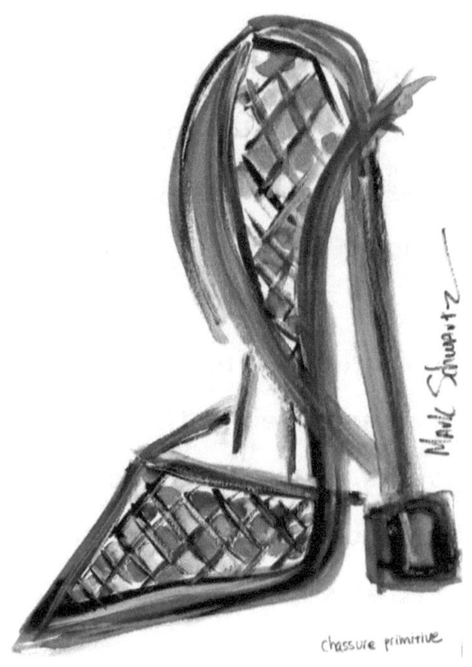

chassure primitive

We might not often think about it, but there is great joy in our daily walk with God. There is more in our daily relationship with God than going to church on Sundays. Our daily walk starts the moment we set our feet on the floor first thing in the morning. Our walk with God isn't meant to be accidental. It's meant to be as intentional as our prayers, our faith, and our desire to pursue His presence. It is as intentional as making sure your shoes match before you leave your home.

When the alarm goes off every morning, God has assigned your angels to be ready and to wait to hear what is in your heart. They may know how to help you not only get through the day but also walk with victory.

Recently, I was having a conversation with my twenty-eight-year-old daughter. That morning, after again watching the YouTube video from Kalina Silverman's TED Talk, "How to Skip the Small Talk," we had a profound conversation. I could hear in her voice how Kalina's question "What would you do if you knew you were going to die tomorrow?" had touched her heart.

She shared from her heart a few profound points. The first one was that she too, like Kalina, struggles at times with feeling alone. Her second point I share in future chapters.

"I do struggle with feeling lonely sometimes, but I don't think it's just me, Mom," she said. "Most people my age feel the same way. When we talk, we all say the same thing," she continued. "We feel like we were given dreams and aspirations when we were growing up, but now that we are adults, we live in a country where the reality of what is happening at all levels—politically, socially, and so on—has not allowed open platforms for those dreams and expectations to grow."

We continued to talk about that for a little while, and as I listened, what I heard her say was she felt unconnected. "Unconnected"—that was her word.

"Mom, I feel unconnected," she said.

When I heard that, I thought, *what an interesting word to use*, so I asked her if she meant "disconnected."

But as she continued to speak, it clicked. "Yes, that's the word: unconnected," she said.

Because we often have spiritual conversations and I know she is a spiritually sensitive soul, I asked her if she feels lonely when she is intentionally spiritual.

After a brief sigh, she said, "No, I don't feel lonely or unconnected when I'm intentionally spiritual."

"When do you feel unconnected and lonely?" I asked.

"When I'm not intentionally spiritual—that's when I feel lonely and unconnected," she said.

"Unconnected" and "disconnected" might seem similar, but they have subtle differences, important differences. Being disconnected means there's a broken connection. There is nothing more frustrating than picking up your cell phone thinking it's fully charged to find out the charging cable is broken, the phone didn't charge, and your battery is almost dead. Being disconnected from God and our spirit means that our connection to God is broken no matter how much we may think we are plugged in. When we're not connected to our spiritual nature, we are inevitably also disconnected from God.

How many of us believe that going to a certain building at a certain day or time of day is what connects us to God? Yet that's what most of us do when we don't understand the spiritual aspect of our relationship to God. Although there is nothing wrong with going to church, I'm grateful to live in a country where I get to fellowship and congregate.

Being unconnected reminds us that we were once connected. Unconnected refers to something that is not joined that ought to have been originally. It's like connecting the charger to the phone but not plugging it into the electrical outlet.

Most of us live unfulfilled, unhappy, waiting for something or someone to fill that void. But we're not sure what that something is, so we fill up the void with shallow things meant to give us temporary enjoyment. Or we try to fill that void with vices like drugs, alcohol, sex, relationships, money, or a career. Deep down, we know that there is something missing, but we're not sure what it is. Something deep inside leaves us unsettled, knowing something is missing, knowing that when we see it and when we hear it, we'll know it is what we are seeking.

In our mind, we split the world up into people who have everything and people who have nothing, forgetting that we are all people, nonetheless. People who walk around with broken hearts on the inside but continue to get up and go to work every day. Have you ever felt unconnected and alone?

So here was my question to my daughter, and I'm also asking you this today: Would you for one moment entertain the possibility that perhaps you are unconnected or disconnected spiritually from God? Not only unconnected and disconnected from one another but primarily unconnected and disconnected from our individual spiritual-identity powerhouse first.

Connecting spiritually sounds like too easy a solution, and where in the Bible did Jesus ever make that statement, you might be thinking to yourself.

In Matthew 5:3 (NKJV): "Blessed are the poor in spirit, for theirs is the kingdom of heaven." This is the very principle Jesus was. The Greek word for blessing is *makarios*, whereas the Strong's Concordance definition describes it as "happy, blessed, to be envied."

Why would God, who went to the extent of sending His beloved son to pay for our sins through the crucifixion, use our brokenness to bless us?

Because He is the God who created us whole. Nothing broken, nothing missing. He is the God who goes to the brokenhearted and gives them entry to His kingdom. He says to you today, "I know your heart is broken, and I have a cure to heal your heart." God will always offer His best to His children. Today, you are being invited to become a precious child of God.

There is no other spiritual journey to God the Father that guarantees salvation except through Christ Jesus. No other religious or spiritual walk can take you there or make that claim.

Doesn't every religion in the world profess to attain some higher potential or level of heightened awareness? It is possible, but not one of them gives you the guarantee of Salvation. Not one, beloved. Most of them offer performance as a solution to inner peace. Or they offer acts of kindness in exchange for God's favor, leaving us with uncertainty, not knowing if God has truly received us or if we made the right choice.

Yet through Christ we have the good news of salvation.

"My sheep listen to my voice; I know them, and they follow me. I give them eternal life, and they shall never perish; no one will snatch them out of my hand. My Father, who has given them to me, is greater than all; no one can snatch them out of my Father's hand. I and the Father are one. (John 10:27–30 KJV)

Chapter 4: Get Your Shoes!

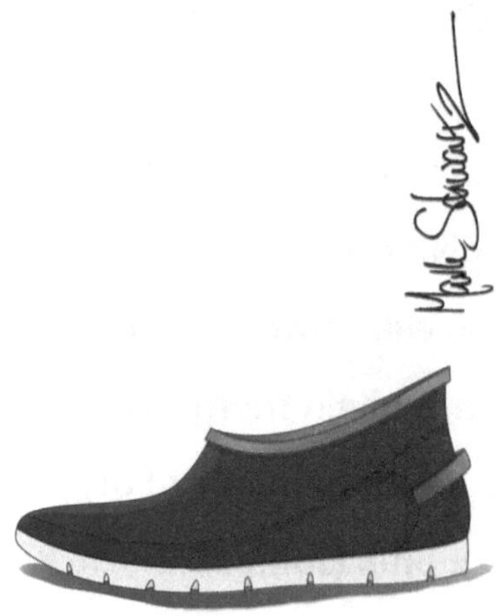

Therefore, seeing we also are compassed about by so great a cloud of witnesses, let us lay aside every weight, and the sin which doth so easily beset us, and let us run with patience the race that is set before us, looking unto Jesus, the author and finisher of our faith, who for the joy that was set before Him endured the cross, despising the shame, and is set down at the right hand of the throne of God. (Hebrews 12:1–2 AKJV)

My grandfather was a very tall man, with shoulders as wide as a mountain, it seemed to me at three years old. He had the most beautiful thick white hair and beautiful tan skin. He was a man of very few words. Most of the family knew just by looking at his face if you had his approval. But I knew I always had his approval. I remember him as gentle and kindhearted. I would put my hands in his, and they would get lost in two of his fingers. He was so tall, he might have seemed intimidating to most people, but I knew him as my Papa. All the grandchildren called him Papa. But what I remember most was that we shared the same birthday. I always knew he was my greatest ally. Whenever I would see him, my heart would leap for joy. The sound of his voice was enough to make me stop whatever I was doing and go find him.

Whenever he was around, I would climb his lap or make him pick me up. One summer morning, I remember playing a game of hide-and-seek with my older cousin Richard in my grandmother's attic. I found a perfect hiding place behind the boxes of Christmas ornaments and winter coats. Trying to be quiet, I heard my heart beating so loudly I was scared he might hear it. So I covered my mouth with both hands and peeked from behind the boxes to see if he was coming. I could hear my cousin opening and closing doors, looking for me downstairs. That's when I saw my grandfather coming into the attic. I saw him walk to the corner, where there was an old writing desk. He pulled an old-looking key from out of his pocket and unlocked the middle drawer. He pulled out a wooden box. He put in the key, and when he opened the lid of the old treasure box, the dim attic room became ablaze in pure white light. The light from the window attic reflected on the coins, and suddenly, it was as bright as fresh snow on a mountain ridge at noon. It shined so bright, I had to squint and cover my eyes so I could see what he was doing. I had never seen so many quarters. *Wow,* I thought. If only I could get a few of those quarters, we could get candy at the corner store. I saw him put in a few more coins and quarters, lock the box, and take the key with him. I remember being in awe at the sight of what looked like an awesome treasure trove.

Later that day, before he left the house, I asked him if he would give me some of the coins he had in the attic. With a loving gaze, he asked me what I wanted them for. I was honest, and I told him it was to go get candy at the store around the corner. That was all it took for him to give me the quarters. The next thing I remember, I was putting the quarters in my pocket and getting my shoes so we could quickly go to the corner store and buy candy.

It was as simple as asking. Our spiritual journey in Christ is just like that treasure—waiting for us to come and ask but never forgetting the intimacy or the love God has given us. Our Christian journey is meant to be experienced with childlike enthusiasm, like the joy I had putting those quarters in my pocket and going with my cousin to the corner store.

We often make it appear as if it's a mysterious thing to be spiritual, when in fact, God created us to live a life in the spirit from the beginning. We do not become spiritual because we learn it somehow. We become attuned and awakened spiritually because that is what God intended from the beginning.

Like everything in life, there will be times of misstep and mistakes. But one thing remains true: as you daily pursue God through Christ, you will be walking in the fullest measure of what God has intended for you. Even before you were born, God had set it in His heart for you to walk in all the best He has prepared for you.

Just as you would put your shoes on before a journey, please remember to be kind and patient with yourself and others. This is something I still always need to be aware of. As we continue to grow spiritually, even though you are being perfected in God's very image and glory, there will be challenges along the way. I pray that the shoes you choose for this journey be the inspiration you've needed all along.

First things first: The spiritual journey and walk we speak of in the book is the spiritual journey that occurs at salvation. The moment we receive Christ Jesus into our hearts, our sins are forgiven. The moment we accept the invitation, we become reconnected to the eternal spirit of the God of our creation.

This isn't meant to leave anyone out. On the contrary, it's God's way of extending an invitation to "whosoever will" receive it. Being a whosoever will myself, I extend this invitation to you today.

By open invitation from heaven, we get to walk in the

promises and the fullness given to us. This is the beauty and the mystery of the cross: That Jesus, without sin, laid down his life to pay the price for our sins so we might have eternal life while on earth. That he paid for our sins so that we might become reconciled to God, the Father, and be holy and blameless in His sight.

To be passionate for a familial and intimate relationship with God through Christ ought not to be boring or dull. To have a thriving relationship with God is to have His light, His love, and His grace over your life. As you seek to know God, He will come to know you. Pursue and seek to know Him, and He will allow Himself to be found and will know you and call you His beloved child, in whom He is well pleased.

So, go and grab your favorite shoes and invite a friend or two, and join us on this journey. I'm looking forward to meeting you and your friends along the way as we move forward together on this great adventure.

Know ye not that those who run in a race all run, but one receiveth the prize? So run, that ye may obtain it. (1 Corinthians 9:24 AKJV)

Chapter 5: Determination

To rise and fall, I rise again. To aim on high but fall
again.

I aim to reach and down again. To go and go, I go again.

To push press thru and start again. Get up and go, I aim
again.

Although I fall, I aim ahead. I will rise up, rise up again.

Despised, chastised, and spoke against. I rise, head
high, I am again.

Will not relent until the end. Press on and on rise up
again. God's power and might first seek again. The
sun goes down to rise again.

Do not stay down; rise up instead.

Reach high up high and aim again. Be free, aim high,
rise up instead.

—Sandra J. Petrusaitis

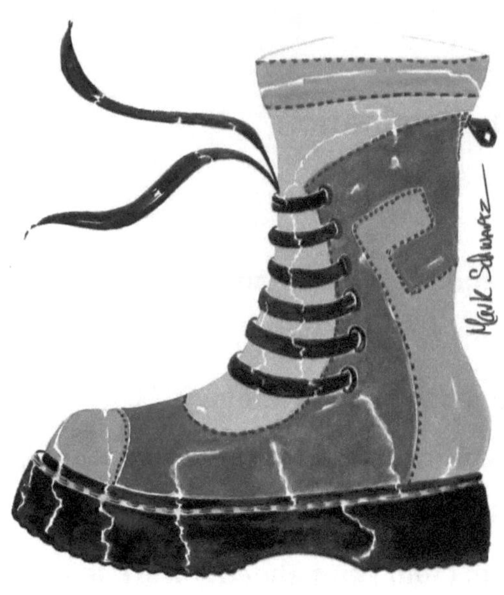

Learning how to overcome your past is pivotal in your daily walk. It's like learning how to walk in high heels and look graceful. I remember when I was learning how to walk in high heels as a teenager. As you can imagine, my ankles could hardly manage to keep me balanced. I would come home from school, and in my room, when no one was home, practice walking as gracefully as possible. I would watch other women walking in their high heels, and I really wanted to be able to walk in them with as much grace as possible. But that takes a lot of practice. I would walk straight, try to pivot, and sometimes lose my balance. But in no time, I got the hang of it, and now don't even think about having to keep my balance when I wear them.

In the beginning, our daily walk with God is similar. It may seem like it's a lot of work, but before you know it, your walk will be second nature.

On its own, determination has no color or meaning. On its own, determination is much like a gorgeous pair of shoes left in their box in your closet. Determination arises from the soul, motivated by selfish or selfless actions. The determination I would like to talk about is the determination attached to faith.

There are no direct scriptures that speak about determination, but there are plenty of Bible stories of women who were determined.

In the book of Esther, we read of her determination to save her people from death (Esther 4:14–16 NKJV), and in a moment of reckoning with Esther, her uncle Mordecai, who adopted her after her parents' death, says to her, "For if you remain completely silent at this time, relief and deliverance will arise for the Jews from another place, but you and your father's house will perish. Yet who knows whether you have come to the kingdom for such a time as this?" It's at this point that her determination arises to carry her through the risk she was created to take. And in verse, she sends a message to Mordecai, saying, "Go, gather together all the Jews who are in Susa, and fast for me. Do not eat or drink for three days, night or day. I and my maids will fast as you do. When this is done, I will go to the king, even though it is against the law. And if I perish, I perish."

In the book of Ruth, we read how Ruth determined to

follow her mother-in-law, Naomi, even to the grave. After Naomi urges both daughters-in-law to leave her and go back to their people, Ruth replied, "Don't urge me to leave you or to turn back from you. Where you go I will go, and where you stay I will stay. Your people will be my people and your God my God. Where you die I will die, and there I will be buried. May the LORD deal with me, be it ever so severely, if anything but death separates you and me." When Naomi realized that Ruth was determined to go with her, she stopped urging her" (Ruth 1:16–18 AKJV).

In the book of Matthew (9:20–22 NKJV), we read of the woman with the issue of blood who, on her hands and feet on the ground, pushes through the crowd, determined to touch the hem of Jesus's garment. In Mark 7:28 (NKJV), the faith of a Syrophoenician woman resulted in her daughter having a demon cast out. Jesus compliments the sheer determination of her faith that He would heal her daughter, "Yes, Lord," she replied, "but even the dogs under the table eat the children's crumbs."

Then he told her, "For such a reply, you may go; the demon has left your daughter." Determination is what will get you up after you fall. Determination will keep you looking forward and aiming high. God is not moved by our need. He is moved by our faith. So be encouraged if today you are struggling. The good news is if your get up and go has got up and went, ask Him to give you the strength and determination to finish everything He has given you to do. He who started the work in you is faithful to complete it.

Like Esther, in Christ, you were also created overcome obstacles. Through Christ, you'll find strength like you never imagined anchored in the truth of His everlasting love for you. So, keep pressing and arise!

Our Spiritual Blessings in Christ

Blessed be the God and Father of our Lord Jesus Christ, who hath blessed us with all spiritual blessings in heavenly places in Christ: according as he hath chosen us in him before the foundation of the world, that we should be holy and without blame before him in love. (Ephesians 1:3–4 AKJV)

Chapter 6: This Is Our Time, Let's Go!

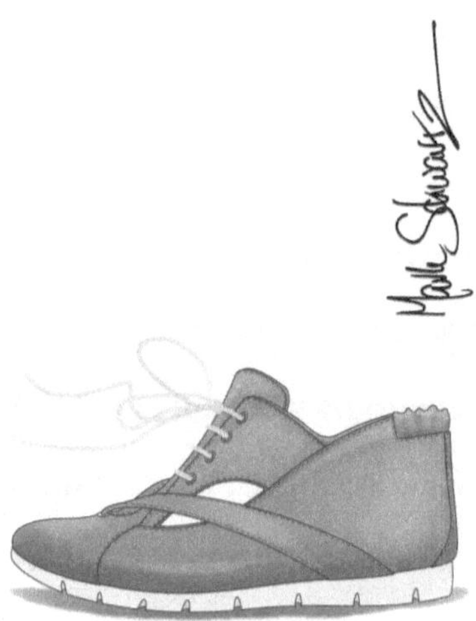

We have this certain hope like a strong, unbreakable anchor holding our souls to God himself. Our anchor of hope is fastened to the mercy seat which sits in the heavenly realm beyond the sacred threshold, and where Jesus, our forerunner, has gone in before us. He is now and forever our royal Priest like Melchizedek. (Hebrews 6:19–29 TPT)

Life isn't fair, but God is always faithful in His word, His love, His mercy, and His grace. It's something I have been challenged with time and time again. I'm sure I'm not the first person ever to tell you that people will disappoint you. But it is during these moments of disillusionment when I need to do the most spiritual walk-talk. I'm not going to tell you it's easy, because it's not. But if God put it in your heart, then to Him, it won't be impossible.

There will come a time when you must be your own cheerleader. The time when you don't want to is when you need to put on your spiritual walking shoes. You must put on your sneakers to cheer yourself to the finish line. Faith is powerful, and a little faith will get you farther than no faith at all.

The worship that rises in my spirit stems from the most pressing and disappointing moments in my life.

People might not see what God put in their heart or the vision and the future He has set for them. You'll reach out to people, and they'll say no. So what, beloved? Get your running shoes on anyway and run the race with perseverance! For every single *no* you hear from someone, or for every closed door, remember, God's *yes* becomes even greater, ever the louder and ever the sweeter. You may not have the connections, you may not be popular, you may not have all of the ABCs after your name. When it comes time for God to make a way for you, nothing is impossible for Him.

What are you waiting for? Now is the time—not the time to see what happens and what you're going to do but, like Queen Esther, to get ready for such a time, as this and walk into your destiny. There has been something in you that has been stirred and compelled to action. You've discerned it, and you've prayed over it repeatedly. You know what it is; however, you keep on waiting for one more day.

Again, I ask, what are you waiting for? This isn't a recent occurrence either.

You know you were born to do this thing that you struggle with. You keep on looking at it from every possible angle. You've looked at it from yesterday's, today's, and tomorrow's perspective for so long. But guess what: it's still there. Mordecai presented Esther with the same truth I would like to pose to you today. *"For if you remain silent at this time, relief and deliverance for the Jews—people of God—will arise from another place, but you and your father's family will perish. And who knows but that you have come to royal position for such a time as this?"* Esther 4:12-14

Taking the first step can be difficult. Especially when it comes to doing something that matters to you. The first step that leads you to the unknown and uncharted places.

Mordecai tells Queen Esther that God will rise deliverance from another source; however, he says that her and her father's house will perish. Queen Esther was orphaned as a child. What Mordecai must have meant is that if she didn't get up and do what she was created to do, God would find someone else up to do it. But all those around her whom she loved, would die not knowing or seeing what God had intended for her.

Alike Esther, in Christ, you are created to display His

glorious splendor—not just for yourself, but all those around you, who are also seeking the truth and light of Christ.

The one thing Esther had to face was the certainty of death. If she did nothing her people would die. If she did nothing, she too would die. However, when you come to Christ, you must die to receive His glorious power. So, no matter how you toss it, if death is eminent, just get up, put your best face forward, and go. Every long journey starts with one step. And when all is said and done, it is better to die trying than to sit there waiting around while those around you perish.

Choose this day. When God says he has come to make all things new, he means everything—from the most complex to the simplest details of your life. In Him, *new* means not having to get up with yesterday's problem but awakening to the knowledge that God is able to do exceedingly more than you could ever ask for in your present situation. He will not refurbish you. He came so you could be made new in Him. Go and get that college application, and fill it out. Call that person who hurt you and whom you haven't forgiven. Whatever it is, just do it! Now is the time, today is the day, and this is your moment. Arise!

> *Have not I commanded thee? Be strong and of a good courage; be not afraid, neither be thou dismayed: for the Lord thy God is with thee whithersoever thou goest. (Joshua 1:9 AKJV)*

Chapter 7: Become

And he said, Draw not nigh hither: put off thy shoes from off thy feet, for the place whereon thou standest is holy ground. (Exodus 3:5 AKJV)

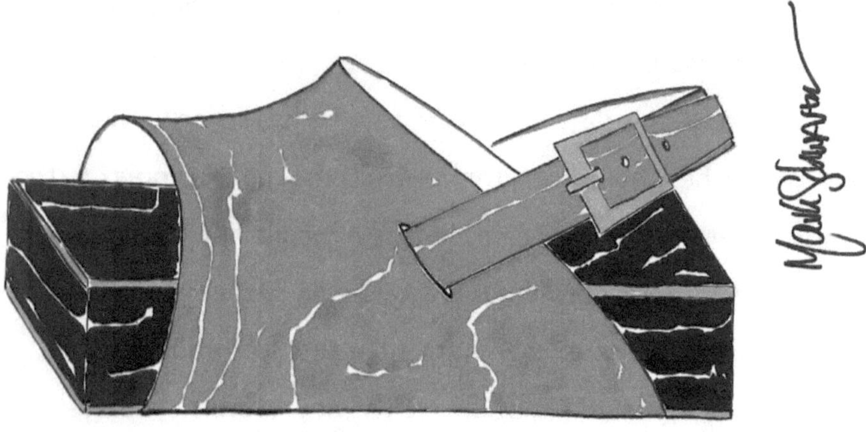

There is something about getting home after a long day. One of the first things I do is take off my shoes and put on socks if it is cold or walk barefoot. I usually take off my makeup and give myself permission to unwind and relax. I'll walk barefoot while I'm home because it's home. I imagine the Garden of Eden to be the same for God, Adam, and woman: a place of intimacy, as a home would be. I can't prove it, but I believe that's why they were barefoot and naked—because they knew they were home and their nakedness spoke of a greater intimacy.

In the garden, woman was taken from Adam's rib. I believe a woman longs for undivided and unconditional loves because this speaks to her creation. Here was God, having put Adam into a deep sleep since He realized it wasn't good for Adam to be by himself. So, having put Adam into a deep sleep, carefully, God took one rib. Then he covered the area exposed with skin.

The word used to describe how God created Adam is *banah*, which means "to build." When woman is extracted from Adam's side, the word used is *barah*, which means "to choose to shape or form." Eden was perfect, overabounding with pure glory.

When choosing to shape and to form woman, God made sure he had no distractions. This is the first father-daughter moment. A father forming, choosing to shape his daughter, purposefully molding and planning her life and her future. In the purest environment, He gave her His undivided attention. Perfectly, he created woman, his daughter, without interruption. He chose every curve and every beautiful part in her to reflect His exact glory. I can just imagine how, while shaping her mind, strong, smart, and complex, He knew the insights and depth of her vision, how she would guide with wisdom and direct and counsel with truth and foresight.

How profoundly beautiful He created her eyes to see beauty in all things. How He created her heart to be as strong and fierce as a lioness yet as gentle as a dove and purposed as a gazelle. How He created a womb that would know the beauty of life and giving life. A true likeness of His very being, in her, he gleaned the hope of redemption, and in her hands did He give her the ability to bless all she would touch. Then when He'd finished choosing to shape her in His image, and he saw her as she ought to be, radiant and glorious, He walked her, as in a wedding procession. And with every step closer to Adam, He knew He would have to let her go. How delicate and precious He had created her to be, and now gave her to Adam as the first bride. So radiant and beautiful was she that one look at her and Adam, with pure joy, accepted her to become one with him.

Bone of his bone and flesh of his flesh. My imagination takes me to that moment. He would have to give his beloved daughter to this man, but he'd also give him the task to care for the garden. Now He gives His beloved daughter to this man. He gently takes her delicate hand and gives it to Adam.

They look at each other for a moment and bask in the joy and awe of the union between them. I suppose a tear made its way to the corner of His eye as God looked at woman's countenance, beaming with pure joy of the moment and hope for the future. What His heart must have felt when he looked at both of them. Would He have worried? Did he worry about her care? A loving Father nonetheless, He must have felt his heart full that blessed day to overflowing, as a father's heart is filled with joy over his daughter and hope for her future.

One of my favorite stories in the Bible is found in the book of Joshua (15:13–19 AKJV). Joshua gave to Caleb a portion of Judah. After driving out some of the enemies, Caleb decided to apportion some land for his daughter Aksah by sending out a message to give his daughter in marriage to the man who would attack and capture Kiriath Sepher. Othniel, who later becomes a judge in the book of Judges, is the man to meet Caleb's requirements.

The story continues with Aksah telling her husband to ask her father for additional land. She approaches her father and says, "Thank you for the land that you have given me." She then asks for additional land that has water rights to sustain the land her father had already given them. The revelation the Holy Spirit gave me with this passage of scripture became a beautiful revelation I have kept close to my heart. When God gives you the blessing of a gift, it might not be all he wants to bless you with. We are blessed to be a blessing. With genuine gratitude, we can always come back to thank Him and ask for additional resources to sustain the gift initially given, and the request will be honored.

I believe most people struggle believing that since God has already blessed them in some way, they can ask for more.

It's not that we are only to ask God for things. But we should have the intimacy and familiarity with God to know that if we need to, we can come and ask. If God blessed us with a gift that needs to be sustained, wont he also give us what is needed to maintain the gift.

We often believe that once God grants us a blessing, we should be grateful and not ask for anything else. We often overlook what God is really wanting. What He seeks is a loving and familial relationship with His children. I've come to experience that as an adult child, I have a hard time asking. But how true it is that when a familial relationship is loving, giving or receiving is only a small fraction of the relationship. As a parent of adult children, I often see how difficult it is at times to ask. I can appreciate how often my children want to try to do things on their own without our help. Wanting to exert their independence or wanting to know for themselves that no matter how hard, they can do things for themselves. I believe that in the heart of every parent, or at least for myself, there is a real desire that they come and ask. Because the asking means they have both the confidence that I want to and will help them.

Our relationship with our Heavenly Father is no different. There are bible verses that tell us, we have not because we ask not. If you believe you were created for a greater purpose, then asking in prayer for what is needed for that said purpose ought not be difficult. So, pray, ask and seek out the heart of God, our Heavenly Father. Greater than the love you might have for Him, know that His love for you is so much greater. Imagine that!

Chapter 8: Praying in Jesus's Name

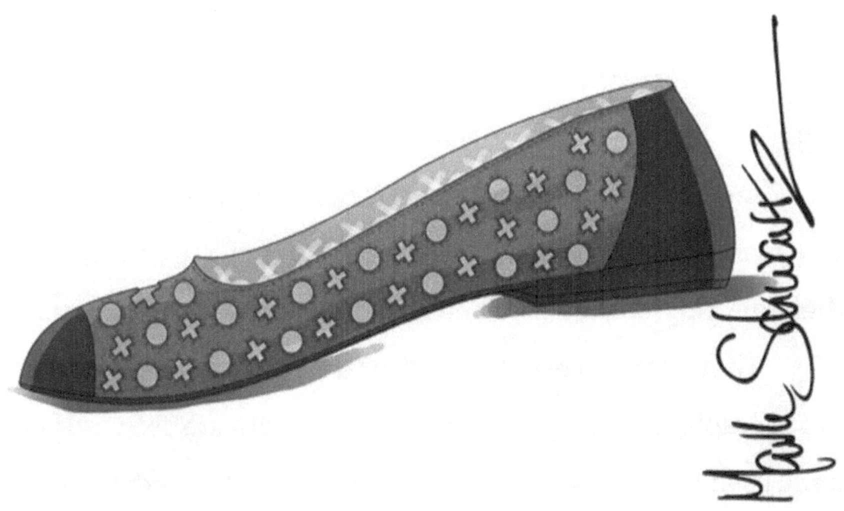

Defiance that pleases God:

To pray in Jesus's name is an intimate act of worship, a legally binding heavenly power, and a defiance pleasing to God.

—Sandra J. Petrusaitis

It's common to hear prayers in the name of God. But when we pray in Jesus's name, we are calling for supernatural divine intervention. When we pray in the name of Jesus, we are approaching the throne room of heaven.

Our petition in His name gives evidence to his resurrection

and acknowledges the power of our salvation and adoption as sons and daughters of God on Earth.

The credited righteousness of Christ is given to us who have been adopted and are co-heirs with Christ.

To pray in His name is not only a powerful and necessary influence in our world today, but it is through prayer that Jesus taught the disciples to approach God's throne.

In Luke 11 (NKJV), we see this beautifully unfold. The story starts by letting us know that Jesus was in a "certain place" when they approached Him and asked to be taught how to pray.

That phrase "certain place" in Greek is the word *topos*, as in topography or a geographical location. There are six words in Greek used in the New Testament for the a single word (prayer) we use in English.

In Luke 11:1 (AKJV) the word is *proseuch*, a term used for when you come into the immediate presence of God in adoration and worship.

The disciples, all being Jews, grew up knowing how to pray at the synagogues. So, what was it that made them ask Jesus, of all things, how to pray? Imagine what the disciples must have seen. There had to be a tangible manifestation of such prayer, because they saw Jesus praying and waited for Him to finish before they asked Him to teach them.

This is the same type of prayer that we have gained as Christians. To pray, or *proseuch*, and to be before God's presence with such worship and intensity in the name of Jesus and the power of the Holy Spirit.

This, beloved, is the legal right we have in and through Christ. We can enter it daily and come boldly. When we pray in Jesus's name, we are also defiantly declaring our legal right and inheritance. This is the meekness and humility that pleases our Heavenly Father, that we as sons and daughters would defy the spirit of unbelief.

Why is it that prayer to God isn't offensive but praying in Jesus's name is received with immediate hostility and resistance? When the name of Jesus is uttered in prayer, you can sense the tension. The name of Jesus is so supernaturally profound that the enemy becomes immediately tense at the utterance or sound of it. Have you ever considered why is it acceptable to use profane words attached to Jesus's name but not with any other religious name?

When reading the Gospels, there are many references to the political atmosphere of the time. There were many conflicting views. There were politics, and there were religious groups. Every group had a purpose and a cause. Then entered Jesus, with no political or religious association, speaking against what had been tradition and convention for hundreds of years.

So, if Jesus wasn't affiliated politically or religiously, what message did He bring?

Jesus came to show us that God is above form and ritual

but that God, being supernatural, was capable of more than what they had come to accept. Jesus came to show us how to reconnect with God, first through salvation in and through Him. He came to pay for our sins by surrendering His life so that we would be able to connect to God the way He was connected to God. He came to teach us that the kingdom of God is a real place while we're alive.

To pray in Jesus's name is inviting the supernatural power of the Holy Spirit to intervene in our daily lives. The reality of God and the power of the Holy Spirit are often debated. But you will start to notice that, as you start to pray in Jesus's name, there is an impact. Sometimes, when you start to pray in Jesus's name, things seem to get worse before they get better. That's the reaction of the enemy, trying to discourage you from praying and calling upon Jesus.

In the early days of my walk, I did not know what I now know: that there is a disproportionate supernatural release of God's goodness when I pray in Jesus's name.

Even when I don't see the evidence of my prayers happening immediately, I have come to learn that, one way or another, God always makes a way, and I will get to see, hear, and witness answered prayers.

I've had prayers answered almost before I finished praying them. I've had to be still and wait for other prayers to come to pass. However, God always answers my prayers.

I stand firm and know He is faithful. The One who

promised never to leave nor forsake me is faithful and true. If He is faithful to me, He is also faithful to you.

Praying in Jesus's name, with confidence, is a gift we receive at salvation. It is similar to faith: on my own merit, I cannot do any one of these things I'm sharing with you today. Neither did the disciples.

Prayer is a discipline that calls for raw authenticity. Initially, it can be challenging to pray to a God you cannot see or touch. Authentic prayer calls for a nakedness of your soul that is counterintuitive. Before doing ministry, I'd pray, but never at the level or depth the Holy Spirit has led me to pray. The more you reveal to God what is truly in your heart, the more He allows you into the deeper revelation of His person.

Looking back from this point in my life, I see there have been times, some recent, where without the revelation of Christ, I would not be alive today to share this with you. I have had experiences where the enemy thought I would be destroyed or led into destruction, but I was protected by the Holy Spirit, only to find that the Lord God Almighty had allowed certain situations to occur to destroy the enemy's work. So powerful is it to pray in Jesus's name that the dead are resurrected. The life I live is a life of a resurrected child of God.

Why would I say that? Because I know that through the darkest, most tormenting times of life so far, I have uttered this most precious name in my prayers. The name that is above all names and has the power to unleash heaven upon Earth. This is the power of praying in the name of Jesus. Because the name of Jesus is known as the name that carries the Victor's crown, beloved. This is our confidence.

Each of these words would express the heart or attitude of prayer while encompassing the aspects of prayer—submission, confession, petition, supplication, intercession, praise, and thanksgiving.

1. *Aiteo*: to pray with an attitude that expects to receive an answer from God.
2. *Deomai*: to plead out of the desperation of urgent need, or to beg.
3. *Proseuchomai*: to come into God's immediate presence in adoration and worship, as in one praying, seeking God's face.
4. *Euchomai*: a pious prayer, or to make a vow.
5. *Deesis*: urgent supplication made exclusively to God.
6. *Proseuche*: a prayer brought to God in an attitude of adoration and worship.

Of all the gifts, prayer is the most powerful and effective. To pray the way Jesus taught the disciples is to say a prayer that comes from your heart. The seven Greek words are the heart or attitude in the prayer that flows out of the heart. For instance, a *deomai* prayer is a spontaneous and authentic prayer that cries out to God in our most desperate time of need. It is not a rehearsed or ritual prayer but a prayer of desperation in a time of suffering and need. Powerful prayer spoken in Jesus's name is devastating to the kingdom of darkness.

Living Daily in the Spirit of God

We are Abraham's seed, through faith, and we get to live in the righteousness and goodness of Christ.

God is pouring out His Spirit right now. All you need to do is walk into your local food store and check out some of the flyer's magazines, books, or newsletter boards to see what I'm talking about.

Often, I hear teachings or preaching that say, "You probably aren't as important as Jesus is to have the enemy come to you." But the truth is that if you are important enough for Jesus to have given His life for you, you are most certainly important enough to become a target to the enemy.

When we hear that taught, we put their spiritual guard down, giving the enemy the upper hand. It would be like saying, "I know you have a brand new car, but you're not important enough for anyone to steal it, so you can leave the key in the ignition and the doors unlocked."

There is nothing more beautiful than living in the Spirit of Christ. Jesus surrendered His life that we may walk in the beauty of the fellowship with our Heavenly Father through the Holy

Spirit. However, as beautifully sublime as it is, there needs to be an awareness of a real enemy.

I became a born-again believer at the age of eighteen in the basement of a local Catholic church in my community. When I was in my late teens, you'd most often find me with my grandmother and my mother attending Mass and church events. My mother and grandmother regularly attended Friday-night prayer at the local Spanish parish. I remember receiving the Holy Spirit and being baptized in the Spirit. In lay terms, this means I received the Holy Spirit and spoke in tongues.

It was many years later, in my thirties, when I started attending a non-denominational church, that I began to understand what receiving the Holy Spirit really meant.

It was at this time that I was drawn to learn the Bible and what it meant to live a life in the spirit. The moment I began to study and learn the Bible, my spirit began to grow. It was then that I developed a hunger for the things of God.

I have no shame sharing with you that, for many years, my family and I were a target. There is no weapon the enemy can use to destroy you, since we have already attained victory through Jesus Christ and the power of His resurrection. However, the enemy preys on the ignorant and naïve children of God.

The truth is you don't have to be afraid of the enemy, but you need to be aware that he hates the children of God. It's not personal. He doesn't care about you.

Staying ignorant of your spiritual inheritance through Christ is what the enemy is after so he can steal what legally belongs to the children of God.

He doesn't want you to understand your spiritual inheritance. Because when you become aware of who you are as a child of God and your spiritual inheritance, you can boldly enter into the kingdom of God. And if you enter into the kingdom of God, which is the kingdom of light, the kingdom of darkness is overtaken by the light of God in you.

Once thing is certain: the enemy is defeated. When Jesus said it was finished on the cross, it was finished. Though the word of the cross is finished and, yes, we walk in total victory, we live in a world where the enemy remains.

Chapter 9: Hunger for Love

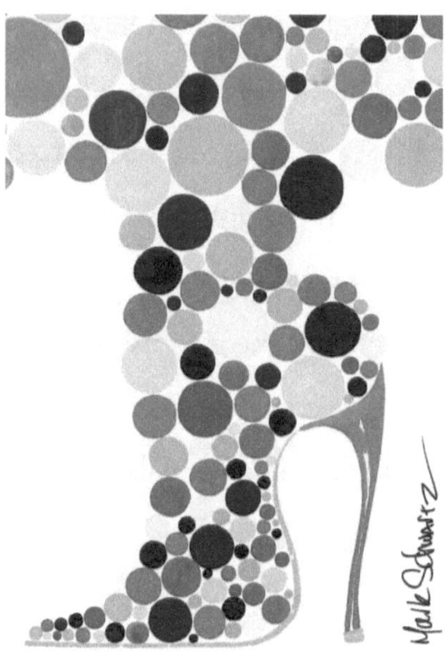

But he answered and said, It is written, Man shall not live by bread alone, but by every word that proceedeth out of the mouth of God. (Matthew 4:4 AKJV)

We are living in a time of an unknown famine. We eat and remain hungry. We drink and remain thirsty. We live thirsty for truth, hungry for justice, and believe the lie that we're lost.

There is a famine that is consuming the soul of an ageless and faceless generation for the word of God.

Recently celebrating my twentieth wedding anniversary, I

was met by a glorious day, just as glorious as my wedding day. The sky was blue, and not a cloud lingered in the sky.

"Hey, let's watch our wedding video. It's been a long time," suggested my husband while I was making lunch in the kitchen. We hadn't seen it in years. While eating lunch, we reminisced about the flowers arriving late. How beautiful my round bouquet of deep red roses filled the air with the divine scent of roses. Walking to the living room, he pulled out a DVD to insert into his laptop.

When we got married twenty years earlier, the latest technology was cable television, alphanumeric pagers, and VHS video players. We have some beautiful photos, but we put so much more emphasis on the video. Nowadays we're so accustomed to how quickly technology is changing that we don't often give it a second thought. Worried that the tape would break or we wouldn't be able to view it, I finally had the VHS videotape digitized into a DVD. An obvious sign of the times.

As we sat there, the first thing we commented on was our youth. We laughed at how we thought we were so mature and so adult. We looked at friends and family with a greater sense of awe and love. As we sat next to each to other to watch the video, it was as if we were once gain experiencing the emotions of that day, yet much more profoundly.

We were both blessed to see Reverend Stevens, a very special man to both of us. He gave us wise council, and every time we met with him before the wedding (a premarital requirement), he asked us tough questions but with such love and tenderness. He was not a man to hold back but never overbearing in his delivery.

We replayed the scenes with my grandmother, and our hearts were filled with the joy of seeing her beautiful countenance. My heart grew warm to see her and hear her voice.

All the familiar faces and all the memories of colleagues, friends, and family we still hold near and dear to our hearts. It sounds cliché, but it does seem like yesterday. It was two decades ago. It almost feels as if we boarded a time capsule and landed two decades later.

We replayed the scenes with his father and commented how much we missed him. We shed a few tears but knew that, one day, we would be with them in heaven.

Then there was Father Simon, a Jesuit priest and one of my professors from college, who will always hold a very special place in my heart. He gave both his benediction over the meal we would share and also a blessing over our marriage. Those beautiful words have never left my heart since the first time I heard them. Every time I hear that benediction, my spirit receives every single portion from heaven. His benediction wasn't only incredibly beautiful, but it was received by and moved my heart.

Before him, I'd never heard anyone speak like he did. Before him, I'd never met anyone like him. But to see him and speak with him gave you such an incredible sense of joy and peace, because it was his Spirit, the Christ in him, who spoke.

In that benediction, he spoke of the beauty of food and why God had created food. How, though for nourishment, God had also sent His son, who became food, the Bread of Life, so that we might partake and commune with one another. So that our spirit, through the bond of community and peace, might come to the banquet that God has prepared for us.

Love is as essential to the human experience as food is to life. We have the ability to breathe without thinking because of the hypothalamic system, which breathing and blinking automatic responses. Your body has the potential to maintain and sustain itself. In the past thirty seconds, while reading this chapter, you've taken approximately twelve to twenty breaths, blinked approximately ten times, and, as you have processed the chapter's contents, had approximately 3,472 thoughts per minute.

God's initial intention for us in the garden was for love to flow from Him unto us just as naturally and automatically as our breathing (Genesis 2:6 AKJV). At the fall of man, that tie was severed, and we lost the connection; however, there remains a deep-seated need for being loved, feeling loved, and being accepted. This is an innate human condition.

The need to be loved crosses all social, economic, ethnic, and cultural barriers. Whether you believe it or not is irrelevant.

It is what it is. Just like breathing. Breathing is not a right but is essential for human existence.

In the same way, so is love.

Love is a need, not a right. To be loved, feel loved, and be accepted by others is one of the basic needs for a thriving life and existence. The hunger for love we are facing as a culture goes deeper than any drug, any vice, or any food we can consume.

That's why, in order to receive God's love, you must surrender to it. God created you in an environment of pure love. In the fall, you lost it, but in Christ, you become reconciled to the Father and are destined to walk in it. You can't earn it. You can't buy it. You choose this love or you can reject it.

I'm always in awe at how God—being greater than the sum total of His creation, King of the universe, the one whose hand set the stars in place and created the mountains—chooses to reveal Himself to us, His creation, not just as a mighty God but through Christ Jesus as your Heavenly Father (Ephesians 1:3–14 AKJV).

Beloved, Christ's crucifixion is the ultimate demonstration of love for you. Yes, you. He became the Bread of Life to feed you and me and show us His love. He carried and hanged on a heavy wood cross to show us He carries our burdens. Upon His head is a crown of thorns to show us His constant thoughts about us. And as the crown of thorns lies just above His ears, He shows you that He's always listening for us to come to him. The gaze of His eyes shows that He longs to see us running to Him. With His lips, when He speaks, He shows us that His truth will set you forever free. In His arms and hands, He shows us how He longs to hold and comfort us. Upon His side is the wound that shows He chose death rather than to leave us. The marks on His feet show us that He runs after us, seeking us. At His last breath, He showed that He longs to breathe His love upon us. And when He rose from the dead on the third day, He showed how death itself could not contain His ever-living love for us.

He lived, He died, and He rose to show us how much He loves us all, one at a time. Totally and completely. We're not lost in the crowd of the world. He sees you, and he desires that you also come to know and see Him.

Chapter 10: Eternal Life Starts Now

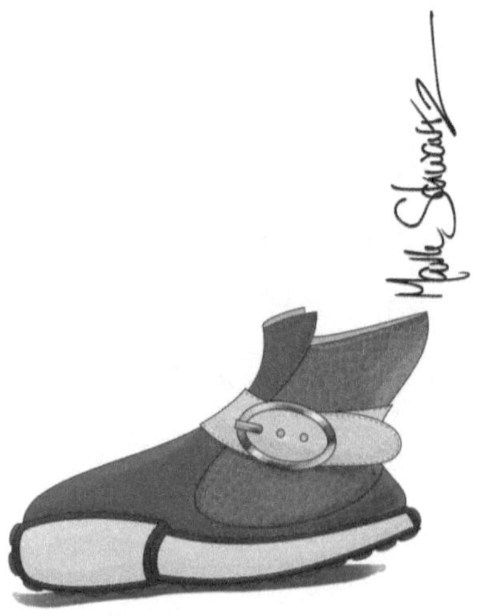

For God so loved the world that he gave his one and only Son, that whoever believes in him shall not perish but have eternal life. (John 3:16 NKJV)

Eternal life doesn't start when we die physically, and our bodies are buried. Eternal life, as we have already discussed, starts here right now, not when you die. If you wait to start your eternal life after you die, you are showing up too late. When you accept God's invitation to become an adopted child through His Son, you enter God's kingdom of heaven. This is where the kingdom of God becomes our inheritance, in and through Christ Jesus and the joint heirs of the kingdom of God.

The kingdom of God is indeed a spiritual matter, a real place. Religion would say that you enter God's kingdom when your physical body has died. You might be asking: What's the difference between being religious and being spiritual? Being religious is the practice of faith in action without the revelation of the Spirit Christ. Being spiritual, according to the Christian bible, is the fullness of the revelation of the Gospel of Jesus Christ. It is not separate from religion but complete in and through the revelation of Jesus Christ himself.

We, although fully human, through the redemption, the cross, and the resurrection of Christ, are being transformed into spiritual beings in Christ's image. And now there is no obstruction or hindrance(sin) that keeps us unconnected or disconnected from God the Father. We are loved, each one of us. Just as deeply and profoundly as Christ is loved. It is an everlasting love, a love deep and profound that He did not hesitate to give up His son's life in exchange for you and me (John 3:16 AKJV). We then have the confidence that we are in God's hand, never to be taken away. We can walk with the certainty and confidence that even if we make mistakes, in Christ, we have been perfected through the God-given righteousness of Christ

Beloved, in you, God created a masterpiece from the very beginning. Living one minute in our modern-day culture outside your spiritual nature will drown out your spirit if you let the wrong influences into your heart, mind, and spirit.

How to live daily in your spirit is a learning process. It is a daily discipline to seek God, learning to walk in His presence, that matures into a lifestyle. This lifestyle requires the discipline of choosing the grace of Christ, freely given yet actively pursued.

Spiritual Identity

In Genesis 1:26–31 (AKJV), we read how God created us in His image and likeness. Triune, three in one, the Father, the Son, the Holy Spirit, not separate or splintered but complete and whole and each a personhood manifesting as One.

You are a spirit first. You possess your soul, and your spirit lives in your body. When you do not understand your triune nature, and the distinct functions of each part of who you truly are, the parts of you that are ignored will always be restless, lost, and unsettled, waiting to be recognized and accepted by you.

The best way I can find to describe our triune nature would be to use our physical body as an example. Having a fully functioning physical body and all its senses. Only recognizing the left side of your body and believing you can only do things with half a body.

It reminds me of a story I once heard of an eagle who grew up in a chicken coop. He had no idea that he came from a powerful species with unimaginable abilities. So, every day, the eagle would get up and do just enough. Just enough to get through the day. Just like the chickens. Just enough to fit in and not be feel different. Until one day, when there was a gust of wind stronger than any other wind experienced at that chicken coop. The eagle saw all the chickens being scattered, but he began to fly and soar. While the chickens were being tossed all about, the eagle expanded his wings, and before he knew it, he soared high in the sky. At first, the eagle was in complete unbelief that he could fly. But now, understanding that he could, he allowed himself to soar as high as the wind would take him. Every moment was more precious than the next, because he had connected to the part of itself, he'd never known. He might not have known what to call this new thing he discovered, but he did know that he had been created to do it. There, that eagle found a sense of freedom and expression he'd never known.

Like that eagle who grew up in a chicken coop, your spirit was created to soar. It's the part of you that soars through the storms of life. It will bring hope and lift you out of the uncertainty life may bring. You have the supernatural ability to fly above your circumstances. It's part of our supernatural nature through Christ. You were created in the very image of God (Genesis 1:26-31). He created you with the intention of greatness and fullness in all you are and in all you do.

Chapter 11: Connect to God Again

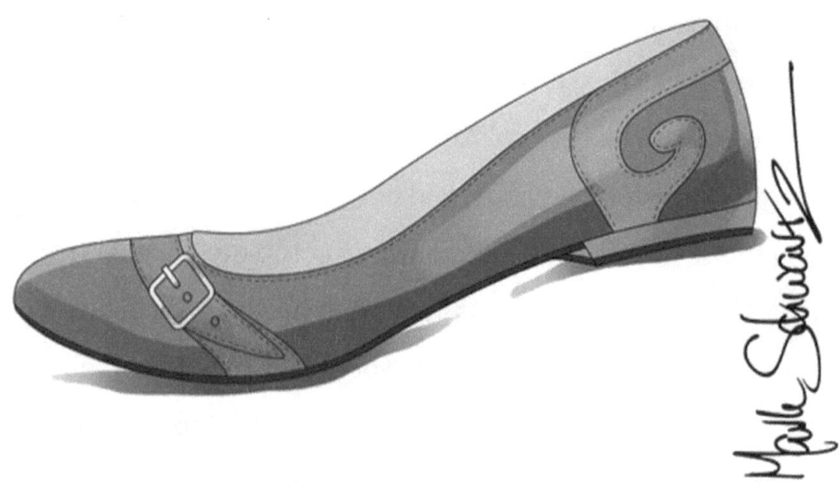

The Lord God is my strength; He will make my feet like deer's feet, And He will make me walk on my high hills. (Habbakuk 3:19 NKJV)

Remember that conversation I was having with my daughter a few chapters ago. Well, here is the second profound point she made: "I have no idea what part of me is my soul or my spirit or my heart," she admitted. "I know when I'm feeling spiritual, but I'm not really sure what part of me that is."

So, that's why we are on this journey together. All the spiritual parts of you that you do not acknowledge or accept become the very parts of you that will always work against you. All the parts of you connected to God are the most perfect parts of you when you become reconnected with God by receiving salvation through Christ. It is in your spirit where you receive the Holy Spirit and through Christ become reconnected, redeemed, and reconciled to God the Father. This was God's original intention for each one of us. We were never meant to be unconnected from God's spirit in the first place.

Our bodies and the distractions of life try to restrain what we believe to be true. Because we can see ourselves reflected in the mirror, we tend to believe that is all that's there. That's it. We're only a physical body, and when we die, the game is over. But that isn't at all the truth or the reality. Since your spirit lives within you, we tend to give more attention to the outside. The Bible refers to this as the "flesh" or "soulish" part of ourselves. It's the part of you that is most obvious to yourself and to the world so it's easy to believe that that's the sum of who you are.

That's because it's the one most demanding of your attention. But we all intuitively know that we are more than our bodies, because we all long for a deeper meaning and connection than just feeding our bodies. We are born wired for and desire to recognize our purpose.

This brings us to a question I hear frequently: Is the heart and the soul the same thing? I've heard people speak of the heart and the soul as if they are the same. But there is a difference. The difference is that the soul is where your personality and is, your possession or what you have ownership over. You soul is what you are ultimately responsible for, and you are not the only one who wants to possess it. More on that later. Let's first talk about the heart and what it is from a biblical perspective.

Your heart is the part of you that has the potential to be loving and receive love. It's the part of you that has the potential to be kind. To be generous. The part of you that houses all your good, bad, and indifferent emotions.

> *God's word is alive and working. It is sharper than the sharpest sword and cuts all the way into us. It cuts deep to the place where the soul and the spirit are joined. God's word cuts to the center of our joints and our bones. It judges the thoughts and feelings in our hearts. (Hebrews 4:12 ERV)*

We have a spirit, and when we surrender our hearts to God, we receive His Spirit. Our spirit that dwells within us now is a place where God's Spirit and your spirit become one through Christ. It's in our heart, where our soul manifests our emotions and processes thoughts. I'm not referring to your physical heart. It's here, in your heart and where your emotions are profound. Where your passion and desires live. That part of you speaks the language of love and loyalty. It is the emotional center of your being. Your heart is where relationships with yourself and the world around you form and emerge, where you get your heart broken, where you fall in love and form lifelong bonds—family and friends.

Our hearts are fed through the meaningfulness of our lives, our relationships, and our contributions to our world. Our hearts were created to be the expression of God's love in the world. We each have a place. Not everybody does the same things. That would be redundant. However, some have a position that has been given to help others who are awakening to the power of God in their lives.

Not everybody is called to preach or teach, but as sons and daughters, a people belonging to God, there is a form of service you have been given, and service is expected.

You might have been given a brilliant mind that will find a cure for sickness and disease. Or you may be gifted with creativity.

The disciples were the first to have been called by. Then the Apostle Paul was called to build and expand the good news or salvation. But God doesn't necessarily do the same thing repeatedly. The God we serve through Christ Jesus is a creative and innovative God. He rules over all things, and everything has been created by Him. He is God the creator of heaven and earth. So, when He created man in His very own image, it was so that we would exemplify and manifest His loving-kindness in all aspects of love. Love has many expressions. In the Greek language, there are four concepts of love. There is the *phileo*, brotherly love. There is *eros*, or sensual love. There is *storge*, familial love. Then there is the God kind of unconditional love, which is *agape*.

There is no greater love than the love of God, and humanity is the ultimate expression of that love. That we exist is a miracle we don't usually think about. And that we exist with the potential to have empathy and to love is the expression of God manifested in humanity.

Our heart is a melody resounding the expression of a life lived with zeal and passion. Out of the three parts of our divine human nature, our heart is as unique as a fingerprint, an imprint that gives glory to the God who created us as magnificent reflection of His very image.

It is our heart that most often reflects God's glory and generosity. When our hearts become fully surrendered to God, the Spirit of Christ within us amplifies the exquisite and glorious nature of God. Just like diamonds, our hearts become brilliant in the light of Christ and His glory.

When we live in the Spirit of God, we all become situated in a position where God, through His Spirit, is serving and living and thriving. It is the ever-giving force that will compel us to compassion and love for one another.

When we believe in Christ, through faith, love and the expression it brings become magnified within us and overflow, provoking that same love and kindness in those around us. The expression of love is as contagious as laughter.

When you think of the function of your mind, you might think, "Well that's easy. It's where I think." I'm not talking about the physical brain. However, your mind is the sum of your human consciousness: your thoughts, your intelligence, your intellect, your memories, etc.

The mind is so complex it is best left for experts in the field of neuroscience to give you a scientific definition. Since I'm not an expert or a neuroscientist, let's agree that the mind is the part of you that processes thoughts, intelligence, and intellect via your consciousness.

But what is most important to know is that the mind is more than where we process our thoughts. Our minds are so complicated, it would be very easy to go off on a tangent. But what I do want to make clear is that your mind is more than a negative or positive attitude.

When we become spiritually intentional, our mind is what is most revolutionized. It's in your mind, your attitude, your belief system, and your perspectives where you will face most of your challenges. There are numerous resources and books on this. Joyce Meyer has numerous books tackling the challenges of faith and the mind. Because of old attitudes and old beliefs, it's here, in your mind, where your faith will be challenged most. How we think, how we perceive the world, and how we start to interact with the world around us are directly connected to how quickly we can break down old belief systems that challenge a supernatural spiritual view of God in our everyday lives.

How quickly we can get rid of old thoughts and empower ourselves, through faith, by grace, to accept and believe that we are spiritual beings, fully equipped to operate spiritually. And that's where faith enters the frame. Faith is the great catalyst. Faith is to the spiritual life what gasoline is to our cars. Faith is the battery powerhouse that allows us to be spiritually intentional. Faith, by its very nature, establishes and fortifies what we believe to be true.

Having said that, let me say that knowing you are a spirit who inhabits a body and possesses a soul is the first step. Knowing is not the same as believing. When you believe that the word of God is true and have faith that you are who He says you are, having a faith that is confident in God's supernatural nature and not your human efforts, you have a rocket that will propel you toward a powerful spiritual life in Christ.

I know your head might be spinning if you've never heard this before. The good news is that spiritual principles are not necessarily taught as much as they are "caught" by your spirit.

Remember earlier, when we spoke about how each part has a different language or a distinct way to communicate? Your spirit is the part of you that perceives the invisible or concealed aspects of God. Your spirit can perceive so much faster than your mind can think.

God is light, and we are children of light. Scientists have known for a long time that the fastest speed in the universe is the speed of light.

I have had experiences where right before I had a thought, my spirit received what God wanted me to know first. Learning to walk by faith is learning to trust whether what your spirit is perceiving is from God. This happens faster than I will ever be able to explain. Numerous times, as the Holy Spirit was speaking to me, I could see what was being told to me slowly unravel around me. God is light, so He communicates at the speed of light. But we communicate at the speed of sound.

It's important to understand that this takes some time to learn and that, in the beginning, you will make mistakes. The level of your receptiveness to the word of the Holy Spirit depends on your level of surrender and trust to Jesus Christ. It's the beautiful choreography of a relationship reconciled through Christ. Salvation in and through Christ is instant; however, learning to walk in faith, by measure, takes patience and the discipline to pursue God daily.

Your daily pursuit of God isn't simply going to church or being a good person. It's not how much suffering you can endure or how holy you behave or perform. It isn't what you wear, where you were born, or how much of the ancient holy scriptures you have memorized.

All these things are not bad either. Let me assure you that, through our salvation in Christ, we *get* to do all these things. We get to go to church to congregate with others for worship and build a community where we are loved and received. We get to do things for one another that most people deem good and kind. We get to bless the believer and unbeliever in the hope that they will receive the gift of salvation. In and through Him, we get to walk upright in the face of fear, hate, and ignorance. In and through salvation in Christ, we get to walk in God's overflowing grace.

Grace, grace!

Grace is a heavenly gift God has given to you. A beautiful gift for you to unwrap. With no fear, you can unwrap this divine gift because your name has been personally engraved on it. It is a gift we don't deserve but which Christ has freely given to those who believe (Romans 3:20–24 AKJV). This is what you seek, what your heart longs for, and what is missing. He has personally written your name in heaven. God does not care what you have done in the past. Your sins have been forgiven. When we come to God with a heart that cries out to be restored and forgiven, He responds with His loving-kindness.

Just as beautiful as the sound of bells on a summer evening is the liberty God has given you from the burden of sins in your life through Christ Jesus. Beloved, in you, God has placed the perfection of His Son. Through you, He has set the testimony of your faith to be a trumpet that resonates the heavenly truth of grace on this Earth. The next time you hear a bell or a wind chime, let that be a reminder of the truth that you are a child of salvation.

A son and daughter who, through salvation, have been given

the precious gift of forgiveness of sin, by faith, through grace, in

Christ Jesus.

Chapter 12: The Spirit in You

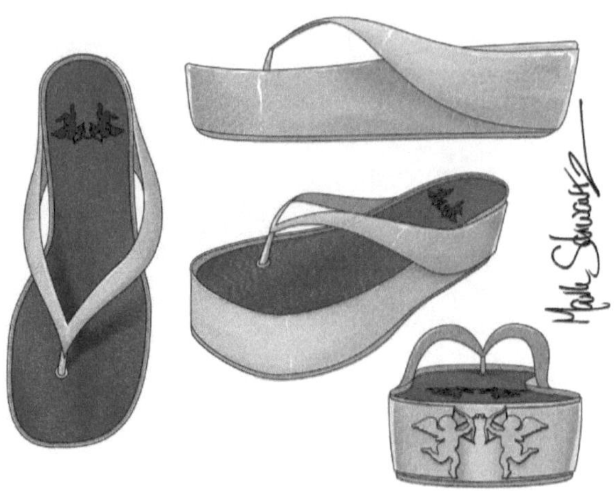

The most neglected and most often rejected part of our being
is our spirit, because we live in a culture that perceives our
spiritual nature as counterintuitive. This is the place of eternal life
within us.

The eternal life spoken of in this verse doesn't only apply
to us after we die. Having a spiritual life is the beginning of your
eternal life from this side of heaven.

Eternity isn't merely a location or a timeframe in heaven.
Eternity, or the eternal, refers to a sphere or realm where God,
Christ Jesus, and the heavenly beings reside. They are not far
away, as we sometimes think or believe. Eternity exists wherever
God's presence abides.

My sheep listen to my voice; I know them, and they follow me. I give them eternal life, and they shall never perish; no one will snatch them out of my hand. My Father, who has given them to me, is greater than all; no one can snatch them out of my Father's hand. I and the Father are one. (John 10:27–30 KJV)

However, in our culture, we think or believe in *chronos* time. In simple terms, it's a linear way of keeping time. We've become a culture limited by our perception of time as it is dictated by our watch, clock, or alarm. But that is changing.

Most of us often believe in time and the following terms: You're born, you live, you work, you get old, and then you die. Game over!

But no, that isn't the truth of eternity. God isn't ruled by *chronos* time. He is above time, having been the Creator of all things and exists in *kairos* time. This simply means that He is, all in all, above all the restrictions and limitations of the time we experience every day.

He exists above the natural daily place we all live from birth. Eternity isn't a fairy tale, a theory, or a concept. It is a place to go after we die. Eternity is not only real; it's accessible to us through Christ Jesus and exists for God's children to live in every day, from the moment we hear the message of salvation and believe.

Eternity is the realm in which the Lord God Almighty Himself is enthroned.

It is far above all restrictions of time and space, making Him the beginning and the end. The Alpha and the Omega. Because eternity has within itself a conceptualization of time, and because of our most predominant concept of time as linear or chronological, we usually categorize eternity as occurring when we die.

But this is what Jesus teaches us in the Gospels. There is a crimson thread of Jesus having heavenly encounters, crossing from *chronos* to *kairos* during his earthly ministry. He did not enter eternity after the crucifixion. He entered the eternal realm through His obedience to the Father while here on Earth. He opened that door so that we too might enter the throne room of grace.

He taught the disciples spiritual principles, and there are many accounts of Jesus teaching, among other spiritual principles, that faith moves mountains when and only when we believe.

We read in the book of John about the time Jesus was baptized. The verse says that the heavens opened, and the Holy Spirit looked like a dove and descended upon Jesus. The audible voice of God was heard saying, "This is my beloved Son in whom I am well-pleased."

We are living in a time where our spiritual identities will become apparent. God will start to pour out His spirit in the way it's spoken of in the book of Acts 2:17 (NKJV): "In the last days, God says, I will pour out my Spirit on all people. Your sons and daughters will prophesy, your young men will see visions, your old men will dream dreams." Initially, it will seem confusing, because evil and its manifestations will also increase. It will seem as if things are getting worse and not better. This is what we call the time of sorrows.

The Holy Spirit amplifies or magnifies everything that dwells in the heart of man. What may have seemed like nothing, now, with the Holy Spirit present, will become exponentially good or not. This is the "dross" or impurities the scriptures refer to. But don't let that scare you. The grace of God is always much more than we could think or imagine.

Grace, just uttering it, brings joy to my spirit. Grace is unmerited and unearned. Grace is understanding that on your worst day, God, in His loving mercy, extends the love He has for His beloved Son specifically to you, beloved.

Many authors and theologians have written about grace. The list is numerous. Among those I have read and heard who have completely changed the way I frame grace in my spiritual journey is Joseph Prince. In his book, he defines grace as a virtue freely given but unmerited and undeserved.

Grace often seems to be misunderstood. I'm not here to tell you what grace is because I am somehow a world expert on the subject. However, if I'm going to share biblical, spiritual insights, it would be impossible not to talk about the power grace has in our spiritual lives.

Grace, by its very nature, is directly connected to becoming alive spiritually. We really can't afford to miss the role grace plays in our salvation and receiving the Holy Spirit. This is because grace is what keeps us humble, reminding us that we didn't earn or deserve God's extension of salvation to us in the first place. We see the beauty of grace unfold in the garden right after the fall. When God went looking for Adam (Genesis 3:9 NKJV), asking, "Adam, where are you?" if Adam had disobeyed God and the price of disobedience was death, why would God seek Adam in the garden? I believe the heart of God was filled with compassion. This was then the first time we saw grace being displayed.

Saved by grace and believing by faith. Sounds so simple. Simple enough that only a brilliant mind can complicate it.

It is that simple. Through faith, and believing God exists and receiving the salvation and the forgiveness of all our sins, we *get* to, through grace, live each day connected to God through our spirit.

That the reality of grace is what compelled God's heart and why grace was extended to use through Christ.

But now the righteousness of God has been manifested apart from the law, although the Law and the Prophets bear witness to it—the righteousness of God through faith in Jesus

Christ for all who believe. For there is no distinction: for all have sinned and fall short of the glory of God, and are justified by his grace as a gift, through the redemption that is in Christ Jesus. (Romans 3:21–24 NKJV)

Chapter 13: Joy Is a Gift We Get to Unwrap

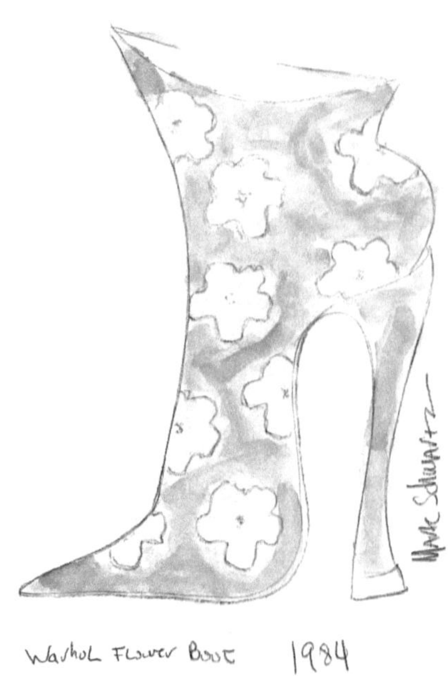

*Now may God, the inspiration and fountain of hope,
fill you to overflowing with uncontainable joy and
perfect peace as you trust in him. And may the power
of the Holy Spirit continually surround your life with his
super-abundance until you radiate with hope! (Romans
15:13 TPT)*

Here I am sitting at my computer, writing about defiant joy and
battling a depressive mood. When I opened my eyes this morning,

the sorrow and despair were so tangible in the atmosphere. Despair, sorrow, grief, and hopelessness all loomed about, waiting to devour my day.

Having tempestuous emotions and feelings is what I describe as swimming uphill. All waves of hidden shadows and darkness, like an undertow waiting for me to surrender to its grasp, to pull me down until I stop struggling.

This unforeseen yet tangible darkness attempting to devour my every move is not unfamiliar. It has attempted many times to wipe me out, to blot every part of who I am, down to the smallest parts of me, from existence.

If I described what I'm feeling to you right now, it would terrify you. It's overwhelming and so profound that even the thought of speaking seems impossible.

You might be thinking I am being dramatic, psychotic, or both. For too many years, this "thing" has tried to rob from me of what I know is rightfully mine. Joy unspeakable is mine!

Never having been a surface type of person, I want to share with you not only the good stuff but also some of my true struggles. I too have had broken dreams and unhappy endings.

But this one thing I do know: Joy is not like happiness, as we have heard it said. Joy is more profound. Happiness happens to you, and when you pursue it, it can be temporary. But joy, defiant joy, is the kind of happiness that resonates and grows like ripples and waves when you throw a tiny pebble into a lake. This divine gift from heaven is the root of life, freedom, and liberty.

When I was eight years old, my mom enrolled me in St. Augustine's Catholic school. The neighborhood was predominantly Portuguese, Italian, and Irish.

As I remember it, I was one of very few Puerto Rican children in the school. This one September afternoon, as we were getting ready for dismissal, as was customary, the principle announced the dismissal over the loudspeaker, reminding the students and teachers of the weekly activities. One that caught my attention that day was the announcement of Irish dancing. All interested students should go to the cafeteria after the dismissal bell.

I became happy at the thought that I would be able to have a dancing activity in school. I wasn't a popular kid, ever. I may have had times when I thought I was cool, but popularity was never one of my experiences when I was in school. In fact, I was always that awkward little girl who was either too quiet to be noticed or, in my attempt to be friendly, too talkative and just as awkward.

Excited about Irish dancing, I went up to my teacher and asked for a note so my mom could sign it.

"You want to sign up for Irish dancing?" she asked. "But you're not Irish."

"So!" was my initial response.

"Yes!" I'm going to ask my mom, and I know she'll say yes,"
I said. She reluctantly gave me the sign-up sheet.

I packed it in my school bag and was on my way home.

When I got home and walked in the door, Irish dancing
was still on my mind, so I told my mom she needed to sign the
permission slip and I would be coming home late tomorrow after
school.

My mom had the same reaction my teacher had.

"You want to do Irish dancing? But we're not Irish!"

"So, what I'm not Irish? I think it would be a lot of fun to
learn, and I'm really excited about it."

"Okay," she said. She signed the permission slip, and I
packed it away in my school bag with my homework.

I couldn't figure out what the big deal was. I wanted to do
Irish dancing. So what? It never occurred to me that just because I
was a little eight-year-old Puerto Rican girl, I would not be allowed
to participate.

That morning, while putting on my parochial uniform, I
noticed the green lines in the navy blue and green plaid pattern.
Funny how I'd never noticed it until that moment. That's probably
why it's there, I thought to myself.

That day in school, I couldn't wait until the end of the day
for the Irish dancing to start. I daydreamed about it all day, and I
may have even dreamed about it the night before.

Finally, the day was over, the last dismissal bell rang. The sounds of scuffling and the squeaking of chairs being tucked under the desks echoed down the school corridors. End-of-the-school-day sounds. The locking of doors. The closing of drawers. The shutting of locker doors.

The teacher started calling and aligning the students in groups. There was the walking-home group, the school-bus group, and the daily-activity group, in this case, the Irish-dancing group. I was so excited, I could hardly contain my smile.

We walked down two flights of stairs to get to the cafeteria, and there was another group waiting for us to get there. I was so very excited and proud to be there. The teacher taught us some fundamentals of how to do the Irish jig and turned on a portable recorder. That was my first experience of defiant joy, not because I was participating in something unconventional at the time but because I was able to participate with a group of girls. I felt a joy that to this day I can't express in words.

The desire to participate came from an innocent desire to be a part of the group. I always felt so different, so alienated and alone.

There was no way anyone was going to tell that eight-year-old little Puerto Rican girl that she wasn't going to do Irish dancing. I knew in my heart no one would have been able to stop me. I knew the teachers and my mom would help me. There was no doubt in my mind and heart that it would happen.

I still remember some of the steps. Skip one, skip two, skip one, two, three, two. Hop skip, hop jump, hop one, two, three, four. The most impactful part was when we all held hands in a circle and danced together.

I felt as if I finally belonged. It meant all the world to the eight-year-old me.

Defiant joy is having the fierce confidence that God has a better plan for you, that His promises are yours and that every single dream ever put in your heart was His idea in the first place.

Defiant joy is a heavenly gift that needs to be unwrapped amid your circumstances, trials, and tribulations. It's exuberant, buoyant, kindhearted confidence that the goodness of God will always find you.

Defiant joy is the resonating of your spirit with the spirit of Christ that abides in you, beloved. Your one small bell ringing within the resounding bell of God's heart.

When the shadows of sadness or dark clouds cold and gloomy attempt to overwhelm you, remember it is this defiant joy that will pierce through with bright beams of heavenly light and break through a new dawning day. It is the light that shines through and peels away that darkness, that is drawn to you, ironically, because of the Light of God within you. It is merely a shadow, beloved.

Living in the spirit allows you to be defiant and oppose the torment, the sorrow, and the grief with the overbearing power of joy. It may be difficult, but it is not impossible.

No weapon formed against you will ever prosper (Romans 8:15–39 NKJV).

When complete darkness, by way of moods or feelings, tries to overtake you, there is the response of the cross.

We live in a culture that seems to categorize Christianity as an archaic and antiquated point of view. However, the truth is the truth. We may not understand all things right now, but there is truth, and truth doesn't need to be understood in order to stand.

Whenever I'm confronted with overwhelming feelings of hopeless and despair, I've learned to go straight to the root by searching my heart. In Luke 14:25–26 (NKJV), Jesus teaches a powerful principle. He says, "If anyone does not hate his own father and mother and wife and children and brother and sisters, yes, and even his own life, he cannot be my disciple."

There is nothing more frightening than having to confront your own heart, your own attitudes, and your own faults. It's so much easier to try hard to repress the truth. But God cannot be mocked or fooled. We may be able to function for a little while harboring and hiding all that hate. We may even be high-functioning hate-collectors, walking around doing our jobs, being amazing leaders, super-amazing athletes, and outstanding citizens of the community, but this is the truth: hate of any kind but especially hate that is directed at anyone, including ourselves, has consequences.

Harboring hate in our heart toward anyone is like secretly

wanting to rule the world while slowly destroying it. Defiant joy confronts the reality that I'm not immune to hate or being hated. No, not one of us is incapable of hating. When I confront the reality of this potential to hate, I become stronger, I become greater.

So, if we're created in the image of God, why do we hate? Or why do we have the potential to hate in the first place if it's so destructive? That is a question we need to speak about openly as a culture, even as a global community. It might be the only way to address it. But I'm not going to pretend I know that answer. What I do know is that when I face up to the hate hidden in my heart, it becomes reconciled by peace. This happens when I let the Light of God beam ever so brightly where once there was deep darkness.

That is the gold in that scripture. Not that we are all so perverse and must put all things down, including the good things of life. Not that we can't enjoy life. But when I have those very real human emotions, I am not to deny them. I'm learning to come to a place where I can admit them to myself and not let it mean that I'm a horrible person, instead of letting them fester in my heart or bury them like I really want to do sometimes.

How I've learned to reconcile that hate in my heart is by admitting it in prayer. There is only one way of breaking through the level of darkness, which I am now sharing with you. You can't hate someone you pray for.

When I understood that in my heart, my mind, my soul, and my spirit followed.

It takes a moment to confront any kind of hatred buried in your heart from a lifetime of pain, offense, and hurt. But through prayer an instant to let it go and be free from the burden of hate.

We have a blessing in Christ, and that blessing is the life He gave. We now walk in freedom and liberty from darkness of despair. Joy is received. It is a precious commodity in the kingdom of God, a gift freely given to you that no one can take away. With it comes a divine attitude of assurance that if God said it, it is so! If God said it was yours, then it is so! If God gave it to me as heir of the kingdom, then it is mine, and no man, no woman, no demon, no imp from hell, from above or below, or from anywhere can touch it. Because if it has your imprint beloved, signed and sealed from the heavens and sent to Earth just for you, then it is yours. Who, more than the Lord God Almighty, has the authority ? Let them go before the heavenly tribunal. Let them go before the throne of Almighty God and attempt to steal, take away, or delay what God has given to you and your household.

Defiant joy is a legacy-bearing gift that will bear witness to what God has declared and approved for you, beloved. You are so much more than anyone will ever try to tell you. Even more than you know. Walk in the truth of who you are, and there you will find the hidden treasures.

Prayer to receive God's joy:

Heavenly Father, I am sorry for having a bad attitude and feeling hate against that person. Please forgive me.

I surrender the hate in my heart to you, Heavenly Father, in the name of Jesus. Please transform that hate into the peace Jesus freely gave us and which comes from heaven. Thank you for your faithfulness, for hearing my prayers, and for the abundance of your blessings in my life. In the name of the Father, the Son, and the power of the Holy Spirit. Amen.

Chapter 14: From Hate to Love

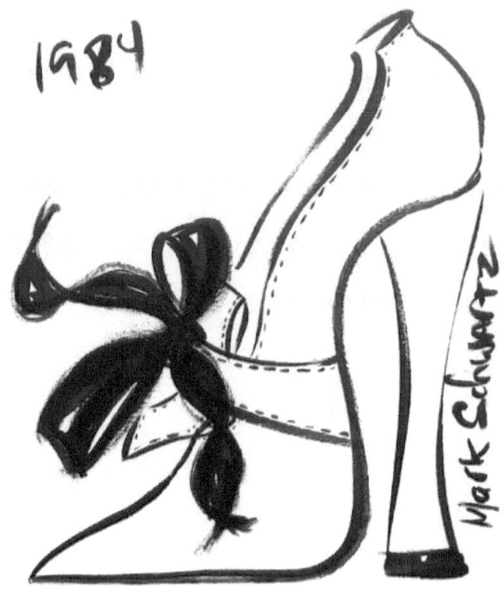

In the chapter of discipleship, Luke 14:26 (NIV), we read Jesus teaching a crowd to count the cost of following him.

"If any man comes to me and does not hate his mother, his father, his brother, his sisters, yeah and his own life also, he cannot be my disciple."

We often think of Jesus as being frail and somewhat of a pushover. The reality is that Jesus was confrontational. He was brilliant in the way he confronted. Nonetheless, Jesus was about being all up in your face.

Yes, He is our Savior. Yes, He is the Son of God. However, that doesn't minimize his impact or the magnitude of His ability to tell the truth whenever and wherever.

This revelation of the hate that we harbor in our heart before we can be his disciple seems counterintuitive. You would think Jesus would have said the opposite: that to be his disciples, we must have love in our heart. But instead, he focuses on the hate. Not that we would have to go and look for some hate before we could become his disciples, but we must confront the hate in our heart. He gets straight to the matter.

I'll paraphrase it the way I initially interpreted it. To me, I heard, "Listen, I know you are all following me because you see a lot of miracles going on. You see how the bread and fish multiply. You see people being healed and resurrected. Don't bother enlisting to be one of my disciples unless you go straight to the hate you keep hiding from yourself. If you can't be honest with yourself, you won't be honest with me, either."

Hearing it that way allowed me to confront myself in a way I'd never done before. I believe this is why we believe ourselves as being broken. Every time we accept hate in our heart, our heart splinters. The hate we allow to fester in our heart will try to destroy love. Just as light and darkness cannot abide the same place. Love and hate cannot. It's light or darkness. Or love or hate. It isn't a "and" but a "or" matter of the heart. Love is always a choice. I'll refer to Christ on the cross. Confronted with hate, he chose to love and to forgive. There is a supernatural ability to love that is a gift that comes from heaven. God is not asking you to do it alone. That's the whole point of forgiveness. When you can't find a reason to forgive and love instead, God will always provide the answer. Jesus cried out to our Heavenly Father on the cross, "why have you forsaken me?" He abased himself. Made himself lowly so that we could through his sacrifice come close to our Heavenly Father in the most needed times of our lives.

This doesn't mean that you must go to the people you hate and tell them how much you hate them. On the contrary, confronting the hate in your heart is being able to come into prayer and reveal the hate so that you can let it go. We will never set ourselves free from the things we don't acknowledge. The things we don't acknowledge will continue to grow like a bitter root, trying to destroy.

It's through the Holy Spirit how we let go of hate in our heart and through prayer how we turn to God and receive help. There is power and freedom through Christ when we are honest with ourselves about the hate we may harbor in our heart. It's time to let go of all that hate that has kept you from fulfilling your purpose and destiny. Were God is sending you, hate cannot come along.

"Forgive us our sins, as we forgive those who sin against us. And lead us not into temptation." Luke 11:4

Chapter 15: Learning to Accept Yourself

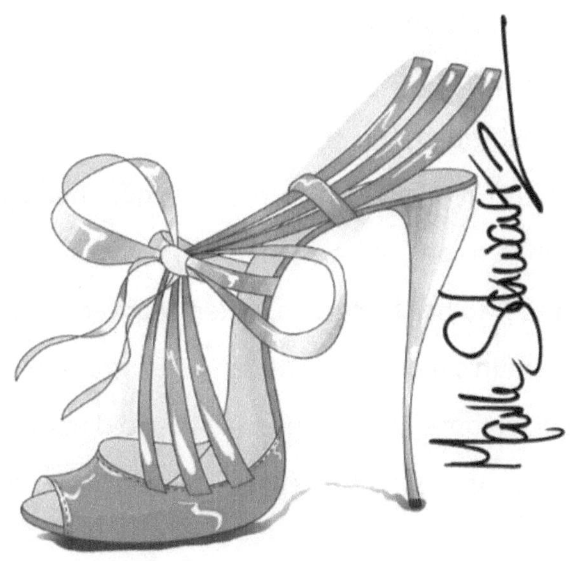

Life shrinks or expands in proportion to one's courage.

—Anais Nin

There is a restless uncertainty in the walk of people who do not feel accepted. This is how I imagine Esther felt. In the book of Ester, in the Old Testament, we read the story of young lady who suddenly became an orphan in the care of an uncle named Mordecai.

Recognition is the affirmation of worth, talent, and effort. Coming from parents, recognition is as valuable as gold. It means that you are accepted and recognized. Even the smallest actions and words can suddenly seem grander when your father praises you or points out your achievements to others. However, when you no longer have your father to guide you and direct you, it is useful to have someone like Mordecai, who recognized and accepted Esther as his daughter.

Notwithstanding the importance of a father's role, there is something powerful about Mordecai's role in Esther's life. Esther chose to continue to be guided by him and honor him as she would have honored her father. So, when Mordecai sent her the message of Haman's plan to kill the Jews, he strongly reminded her that for such a time as this Queen Esther did her God place her in the palace. An orphan Jewess in the palace and no one she could confide in.

Now she had to speak to King Xerxes, but she had not been invited into his court. And to go before the king without an invitation carried the penalty of death. What a horrible time this had to be for her. Her closest of kin was in the outer courts of the palace. With no one to turn to, she surrendered to Mordecai's leadership once again. From the beginning, Mordecai had advised her she not use her Jewish name but instead to take a Persian name. Now he advised her to go to go before the king and plead for her people, the people Haman sought to annihilate. There was no guarantee. She would surely perish along with all the Jews. If not, going before the king uninvited and exposing herself as a Jew would surely bring her death.

Either way, she would go. And if she perished, so be it!

She took her handmaidens, and for three days and three nights, they fasted and prayed along with all the Jews in Persia. It was a deeply somber time. For those three days, even the sun was held behind the dense gray skies, which seemed so thick and heavy. The palace halls and corridors seemed cold.

On the third day, Esther put on her royal robes and stood in the inner court of the palace, in front of the king's hall. The king was sitting on his royal throne, facing the entrance (Esther 5:2 NIV).

My imagination envisions Esther's supreme yet delicate beauty and the deep humility of the moment, knowing that she was taking her life in her hands.

Moments before she stood in the inner court of the palace, she robed herself in the splendor of the royal garments. Not hers but of the king of Persia, King Xerxes. They were made of the finest threads, dyed to regal specifications, and loomed by the finest hands in the land. Once the exquisite fabric was ready as tapestry, it would be sent to the royal seamstress in Persia for the dressing and adorning of the royal family.

How I imagine Esther reverently running her hands through the robes, feeling their softness and admiring their majestic beauty. Perhaps she thought this might be the last time she'd feel these robes since going before the king without an invitation was against the law and punishable by death.

She had resolved to go before the king three days earlier, at the request of her uncle Mordecai, who had raised her when both her mother and father died. Her last message to all the Jews and her uncle was "And if I perish, I perish."

She walked down the long corridor towards the inner court, radiant with beauty and regal in posture. It's the same corridor she entered the day she first entered the king's palace. She had to be prepared for six months with oils and six months with perfumes before being allowed in the presence of the king. It seemed like yesterday, and now she walked those same corridors as queen for the last time.

She saw the entrance to the king's court. Still having the opportunity to turn back, she pressed forward without thought. In an elegant stride, she walked tall and determined to execute her plan. In the few steps she had left before the king could see her standing at the door, he heard someone approaching. Footsteps echoed, delicate in stride yet firm in strength.

Counting every moment as her last, she endearingly thought of the king and how his presence gave her total joy, how he had received her in his chambers with such warmth and such love.

With each defined stride and step, the tension on her face melted, exposing her love for King Xerxes, the one person in the entire palace with whom she had always felt safe. In his arms, no harm would ever come near her. As she reached the court, her countenance was radiant as her heart beat uncontrollably with both fear and hope. Fearful this might be her last moment alive but hopeful to see the king and feel safe in his arms one last time, she appeared just as regal and majestic as the regal robes upon her. She remembered how they had first met and how scared she was. She thought she would die back then. "I really love the way his laughter echoes through the palace corridors," she thought. She never really knew where he was, but hearing the sound of his voice always made her feel safe. That thought took her to the summer night when they ran down those same corridors. Since it was dark, King Xerxes would trick her into thinking he was elsewhere. Then he would emerge from the shadows and frighten her. She would scream, frightened, and he laughed so loudly the people down in the village could hear him, and they started laughing too. Soon, it seemed the whole palace, the palace courts, the palace guards, and the village laughed that whole beautiful summer night.

For a moment, she remembered the king's loving embrace, and her love rose to adorn her eyes.

At the courtyard, she stood in all her majesty. Radiant and beaming, fearful, hopeful, and fearless all at once.

The king was sitting on his royal throne in the hall, facing the entrance. When he saw Queen Esther standing in the court, he was pleased with her and held out to her the gold scepter that was in his hand. So Esther approached and touched the tip of the scepter. Then the king asked, "What is it, Queen Esther? What is your request? Even up to half the kingdom, it will be given you." (Esther 5:2–3 NIV)

Like Esther, you too were created to be regal in all your glory. In your mother's womb did He form you. And your purpose and destiny were also created within you. Consider the timing of your birth, you could have been born at any other time in history, but you are here and have been created with the purpose to rule and reign. You are not ordinary. Every part of you knows it. Your struggles have brought you into the extraordinary. You were created for such a time as this. But you might think your situation is more like Cinderella's than Queen Esther's. The difference is that Cinderella did not have a loving Heavenly Father to love and protect her. But you do. You have a loving Father who has promised, through his Son, Christ Jesus, his everlasting love. You are accepted in and through Christ. You are acknowledged, and He knows you by name. You are both accepted and known by our Heavenly Father. He has written your name in His nail-pierced hands. In Him, you will always be known. In Him, you will always be loved. In Him, you are always accepted.

Chapter 16: A Bond Unwavering

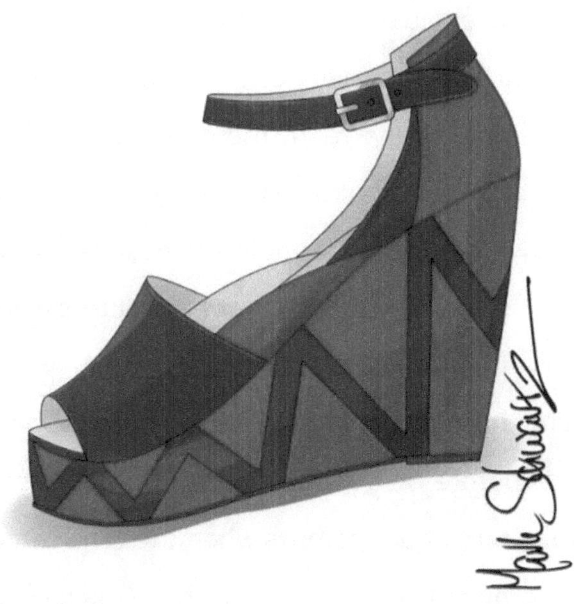

One of the most courageous things you can do is identify yourself, know who you are, what you believe in and where you want to go.

—Sheila Murray Bethe

When my father-in-law was diagnosed with Alzheimer's, it was devastating to the whole family. I had to put on some heavy-duty shoes. When we found out we were all sad; however, in the beginning, it wasn't bad at all.

One day, my husband received a call from the hospital informing him that his father was in critical condition and probably would not live past the weekend.

We went into prayer and knew that we had to help his mother by coming along with her to take care of him. Jack was a retired police officer and a very bright man. He had an even-keeled temperament. I have many memories of Jack being reserved in his comments but always happy to join in and laugh at a joke. That day, when we both got to the hospital, we found none of that. We found Jack quiet, and what the doctors were saying was very worrying.

Both my husband and I had talked about caring for our elderly parents before we got married. We both agreed to help each other take care of our parents when the time came. Now the time had come to take care of his father. God had somewhat prepared us for this moment, even though we'd hoped that our parents would live long, healthy lives.

Because our children were grown, we made the dramatic decision to move into his parents' home to help his mother and father. I stopped working to provide full-time support and be a caregiver. Although I had experience working in the community and being an advocate, nothing could have prepared me for what came next.

If I said it was easy, I would be flat-out lying. It has been one of the hardest things I've done. However, that experience with Jack left an indelible print on my heart and my spirit.

It was very difficult to communicate with Jack after he came home from the hospital. He didn't talk for about two months. As a result of the disease, he was often confused. Worse, he didn't know who we were.

The scriptures teach us that we are a spirit who lives in a body and possesses a soul. My first instinct was to always speak to his spirit. Every time I spoke to his spirit, he responded. We learned to communicate with him in ways that other people couldn't.

Though our body may betray us, our spirit remains the same.

By trial and error, we learned to communicate with him using his love languages. He loved to laugh, so we always joked with him. I loved hearing him laugh. He loved hugs, so we hugged him often. He loved cookies, so I made sure we had cookies to give him.

There came a point where we had to spoon-feed him, fully clothe him, and bathe him, as one would care for a baby. I know that it was through prayer and the power of the Holy Spirit that I found the strength, the love, and the compassion to do this. There were all many times when I felt it was too much work. But it was the bond of love and daily prayer that gave me the strength to move forward. Jack went home to heaven a few years ago. But those few years of caring for him were a time when my relationship with God became so much more profound than I could ever express. I learned to lean on the Holy Spirit and God's pure grace.

I also learned to love my father-in-law like the father I grew up not knowing. Even though it may have seemed as if I was helping him, the truth is that Jack gave me the beautiful gift of the father's love I had not known.

> *I have taught you in the way of wisdom;*
> *I have led you in right paths. (Psalms 4:11 NKJV)*

Chapter 17: The S-Word

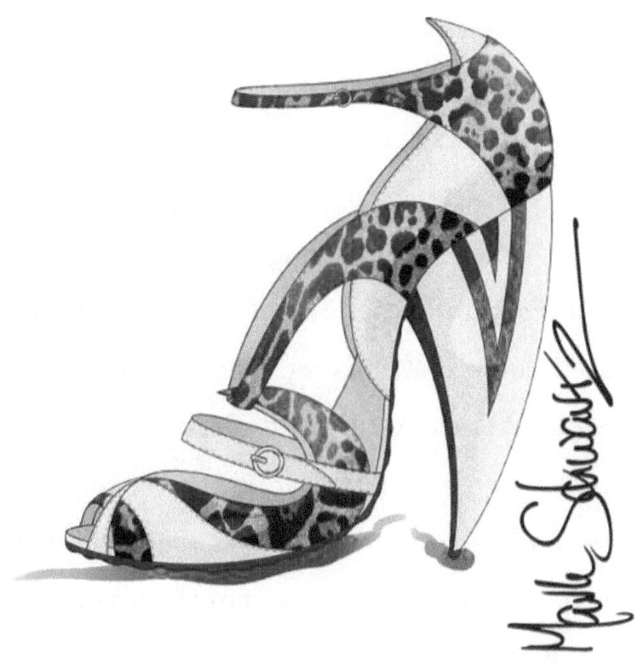

Submission is a challenge no matter how it's presented. Submission is not an end result but rather a work in progress, ever moving and ever changing. The balance is understanding what submission is not.

The first thing to know about submission is that it's not the same as subjugation. Subjugation is violent and destructive. However, submission is neither imposed nor mandated. It is a surrender of the will, a yielding of oneself, in all our parts, to God.

It was years in my walk with Christ before God could introduce the concept of submission to my life, along with other powerful and noble principles.

When I've taught on this subject, I've always gotten two responses. The first comes from women who have no problem understanding submission and receive it readily. Then there are the women who don't even want to hear about it and immediately reject it. I was in the latter group.

Submission has been the toughest issue for me to deal with in my walk with Christ, period. When it came to some experiences, I thought that because I was a woman, I was expected to submit to everything and everyone. The mere thought of submitting myself to anyone or anything was enough to send me into a full-blown hissy fit. And no, I'm not kidding.

In my pre-salvation days, one of my forms of entertainment was to emasculate my male colleagues. One look or a well-timed zinger was all it took to remind them I was superior. Or so I thought. I was rather amused when their ears turned red with embarrassment.

I'm not sharing this because I'm proud. I'm sharing this because I'm grateful that God found me in that condition but didn't leave me that way. In submission to Christ, I was able to find freedom from always having to prove myself.

There is a profound peace in surrendering your heart to Christ.

God first had to lead my spirit and heart to love Him, trust Him, and know Him. It was in getting to know Him that I was allotted with the privilege of truly understanding what God intends as submission.

If you love Me, keep My commandments. And I will pray the Father, and He will give you another Helper, that He may abide with you forever—the Spirit of truth, whom the world cannot receive, because it neither sees Him nor knows Him; but you know Him, for He dwells with you and will be in you. I will not leave you orphans; I will come to you. (John 14:15–18 NKJV)

Submission to God our Father through Christ is an act of love. It is a noble place, a place of high honor. Submission bestows privilege to the one who walks in it. Not everyone can stand to walk in submission, and those who are called and choose to submit must first give up everything.

What I learned was not only eye-opening but also set my mind, soul, and spirit free to submit. Jesus, in Matthew 11:28–30 (AKJV), says, "Come to me, all you who are weary and burdened, and I will give you rest. Take my yoke upon you and learn from me, for I am gentle and humble in heart, and you will find rest for your souls. For my yoke is easy and my burden is light."

Jesus says this because the heavy burden of God's truth

has already been carried and paid in full by Christ Jesus. So, when you become submitted to Christ, you are yoked to His work. And His work, as we all know, is finished. In simple terms, He did the work, He paid the price, and you reap the benefits. It doesn't get any better than that.

Submission as God intends is designed to give us the purest form of liberty and freedom. Freedom, in its purest form in God, is meant to give you access into the laws, principles, and dynamics of His kingdom, hopefully making it clear to you that you're governed either by Christ and His kingdom or Satan and his kingdom—there is no other alternative. However, you ultimately choose.

In God's kingdom, there is but one prevailing and superseding power: love. Submission in Christ is the road by which we are to become reconciled to the ever living and ever-loving God. His blood was shed as a sacrifice so we might enter through His righteousness into the presence of the Highest God (1 John 4:9 AKJV).

Submitting is so much more than the pain of giving up your will or anything else. Submission, just like sacrifice, means giving away the old, broken stuff that will never work. Following Christ without a submitted heart is like launching a firecracker and praying it will become a rocket in mid-flight.

Being a follower and having a surrendered heart is like a

double-edged sword in the hand of a believer: you must have one along with the other for your faith to function properly.

To love God is to follow the principle of surrender and submission. You cannot truly love without truly surrendering your heart, just as there is no giving without a receiving party. Submission and love are powerful forces in His kingdom. Nothing moves outside these principles. In fact, just as nothing moves outside the principle of love, God Himself is love (1 John 4:16 AKJV). And you can truly submit only when you truly love Him. This is because when you love Christ and surrender to him, He is at the receiving end of your love.

Your giving means His getting. And when He receives, then and only then are you reconciled and able to access the One who first loved you (1 John 4:19 AKJV).

In Romans 5:8–11 (AKJV), Paul puts it this way:

> **But God demonstrates his own love for us in this: While we were still sinners, Christ died for us. Since we have now been justified by his blood, how much more shall we be saved from God's wrath through him! For if, when we were God's enemies, we were reconciled to him through the death of his Son, how much more, having been reconciled, shall we be saved through his life! Not only is this so, but we also rejoice in God**

through our Lord Jesus Christ, through whom we have now received reconciliation.

The offspring of your love and submission to Christ is freedom. In 2 Corinthians 3:17 (AKJV) Paul says, "Now the Lord is the Spirit, and where the Spirit of the Lord is, there is freedom." Unfortunately for many, freedom is too frightful a place.

In his book *The Burden of Freedom*, Myles Munro explains that too many people use past oppression to remain mired in hatred and irresponsibility in their lives. He speaks of the spirit of oppression having a specific effect on individuals, communities, and nations. He identifies this effect as a hatred for work, laziness, fear, low self-esteem, selfishness, lack of creativity, low initiative, and distrust of those in authority.

To break free from these self-replicating cycles of oppression, there must be a mental transformation, he says. Paradoxically, freedom requires the need to impose self-control; this requires more responsibility than slavery. The decision to accept a destiny of freedom recognizes the process and discipline that personal and political freedom require, he says.

There was a time in my life when I too walked through this place. We all must face life's circumstances; however, choosing to stay in it is up to you. Being a victim means that something tragic once happened to you. You can be either a victor or a victim, but you can't be both at the same time. There comes a time when you either get out or volunteer to remain a victim. I love the way my daughter puts it: "You're either *on* the rug, or you *are* the rug."

While attending Fairfield University many years ago, I went through some hard times. Here, I learned this victim-or-victor lesson. I was a single mom with three little children to care for and on public assistance.

One day, I went to visit one of my professors, a Jesuit priest who took me under his wing. He always made sure we were all right and would visit us regularly. At this time in my life, I thought I had a close relationship with God. The relationship was not a personal one, in which I got to know and love Him through His word. Instead, I had a relationship based on second-hand information, which might be good for a little while but is not God's ideal plan.

This particular day had been difficult. I was in an abusive relationship and felt I had no way out. I walked up to his office to get advice for his class. When Father Simon saw me, he waved me into his tiny office as he finished his phone conversation. I sat across from him and gave him a big smile. As usual, he asked me how I was doing and how everything was going. I started with my litany of complaints for that day. Just as I started to get into the thick of how horrendous my day was, he abruptly interrupted me.

"Sandra, why are you doing this? Why are you putting up with this?"

"Father Simon," I said in the solemn look of a saint, while

I was thinking, *Poor, poor me,* "If Jesus came into this world and suffered, who am I not to?"

He looked at me in disbelief and said, "Oh, so you think your sacrifice is better than Jesus's sacrifice? You know, He died so you didn't have to go through this."

Those words activated the proverbial light bulb. Suddenly, the spirit of "stupid" was lifted off me. My first response was "Huh … wha … Oh, so you mean I don't have to put up with this?"

He said, "No. No, you don't, and quite frankly, I don't know why you've been putting up with all this nonsense anyway."

This really cleared up my thinking. All those years of frustration and turmoil ended with that answer. When I left that tiny office just a few minutes later, I had changed forever.

Things changed immediately in my thinking. And my thinking changed my attitude, and my attitude my choices. I was very clear and put a stop to the abuse. So, he stopped me from making my life impossible. I'd had it with being on welfare, so I worked toward getting off public assistance. I hated where I was living because my kids couldn't play outside, so I moved.

To be honest, I didn't know how things would change, but I knew I could stop being stupid. When I chose the truth—that the battle had already been won—I activated the kingdom principle of love.

God, in His ever-loving mercy, took care of the rest. So here I am today, only by the grace and glory of Christ. Had it not been for that bold question, honestly, I'd probably still be in the thick of stupidity.

When we suffer, life can sometimes seem tough or unyielding. But sometimes, as in my case, suffering is due to lack of direction.

So, here's my question to you: Is your suffering for the cause of Christ, or are you suffering because it gives you an excuse not to do anything and stay where you are? This is love asking this question.

Chapter 18: Miracles

The LORD my Miracle, The LORD my Banner

(Ex. 17:15) (rendered in the KJV as the Yahweh Nissi)

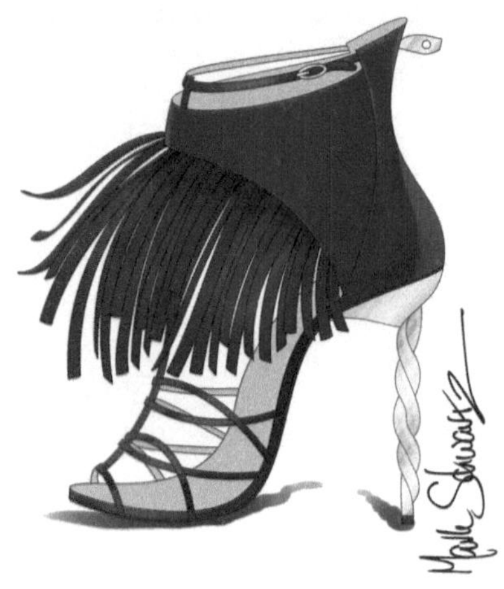

We can only appreciate the miracle of a sunrise if we have stood in the darkness.

Often, I write of what God is processing, pressing and charging within me. By the time you are reading it, each word is heavy and laden with deep emotion.

Every letter in every word represents a pound of flesh, His blood and more often than I care to admit deep misery and frustration along with a childlike wonder. At times tears of miraculous joy, other times uncontrollable tears from the journey of through the valley of the shadow of death seemingly alone and naked with His comfort as my only refuge. And indeed, the only one I'll ever need.

I'm not sharing this looking for sympathy or trying to establish some sort of holiness or self-righteousness. But to share the miraculous work of a mighty God, so graceful and loving, that in our inability to see His greatness, He chooses to challenge and direct away and out of darkness into His marvelous light. In simple terms, he accepts us as we are in every moment, but leads and guides us into His perfect presence that we may share with Him the joy of holiness. Not just a fleeting moment of happiness in strumming an instrument or basking in the simplicity of happiness we express to one another in genuine love and kindness. His heart desire is for us to establish our residency in Him that we may exist in the permanency of His goodness and mercy (Psalm 23:6).

If you're expecting God's miracles in your life to shine like a beacon of light for the world to see and know that the Lord our God is One, then the shadow cast upon you will stretch longer and encompass you farther than expected. You will need to learn how to walk through the darkness.

The joy comes in knowing that though you may not see through the thick darkness that surrounds you, He is there!! Learning to walk in this will anchor your sight to His glory. What you focus your eyes on is the direction in which you will travel.

More than any other miracle in my life, and there are many, I often am stricken with awe at what God has chosen through Jesus, to do in the depths of the soul. It never ceases to amaze me how wicked my heart left to my own human devices could be, at just how mean spirited I could be and the thoughts, words and deeds that can come out of me in a moment's notice.

I'm amazed at how we could be Just like Peter one moment inspired by the Holy Spirit to recognize the Christ, the son of God in your life to be rebuked by Him the next breath. Get out of the boat one minute and walk on water towards our Savior and Lord, then sink while on your way. Swearing loyalty to the death, then denying Him to a little girl. How else would we know that He is loving, if we were not to experience His loving mercy and grace through the darkness of your soul?

It's in the darkness where the light shines the greatest. It's in those moments where your weakness is so obvious not to the world but to you, when God-moments and miracles happen. I encourage you to stay in line, don't lose your battle march. When you think you can't make it, take another step. When you think you can't see it, look higher. When you think He won't pull you out, look out like the watchmen only stopping when you see Him coming.

And when your faith weans and dips, believe in Him anyway. Choose to stand no matter the battle no matter the circumstance. If you want to cry, don't sit to weep. Stand and let the frustration stream down your face. Every step brings you closer to the one that can change all things. Settle it in your heart once and for all. Know that what He has said, He is faithful to complete it. Don't lose sight while in the battle and think the battle is your destination

While in the battle, don't forget that the battle has already been won. This isn't about going before the throne of grace. Jesus already established that we could enter boldly and with freedom to the throne of grace by his death and resurrection. The battle is to remember to speak with authority and with faith the promises of God. Speak them clearly, precisely and boldly. The battle is in speaking out the promises of God when we are aware that we don't deserve anything. As children of God, we don't have to implore for His goodness, or supplicate for victory. As His children, we get to come before Him upright in the Righteousness of Jesus Christ and walk into the Kingdom of God and of Heaven.

Thanking God for all the miracles He has done in your life and for even more to come is the beginning of a life filled with a joy so unspeakable that it can only come from heaven. He promised, and it is so.

Chapter 19: Prayer as a Lifestyle

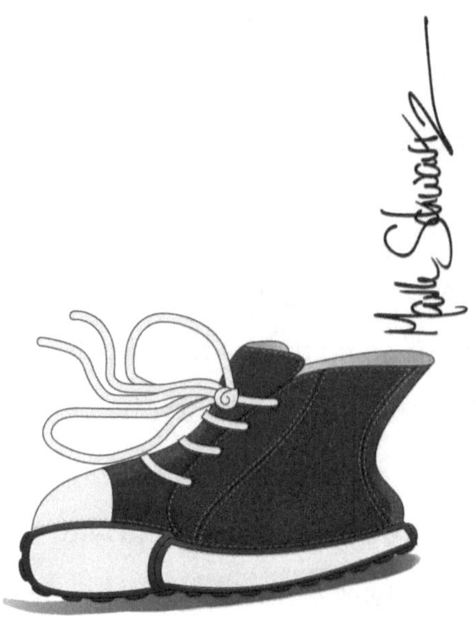

Our prayer for you is that you walk in the certainty that Christ has established you to be a blessing everywhere you go. That with every step you take, you may be blessed to be a blessing. That no matter who you are, you find the love, the peace, and the joy you seek. That as your day turns into night and you lay your head to rest, God will guard your dreams and heal your mind, heal your body, and heal your soul. That when you rise in the morning, you will be prepared to take the next steps in the amazing journey of your life. In the name of the Father, the Son, and the power of the

Holy Spirit. Amen. (Deuteronomy 28:1–8 AKJV, Psalms 63 AKJV, Psalms 103 AKJV, Psalms 61 AKJV, Isaiah 61 AKJV)

Prayer is the most powerful way to communicate with God. Prayer as a lifestyle could mean that you are in constant communication with God. But first, we need to become aware of that possibility by taking that first step of faith.

In the New Testament, we read stories of Jesus walking with his disciples. They were always coming or going somewhere in preparation for miracles. We read of people calling out to Him or pulling on Him in the middle of a crowd, as Blind Bartimaeus did (Mark 10:46–52 AKJV). When he first yelled out for the Messiah to heal him, he was told to sit and be quiet.

The woman with the issue of blood crawled on her hands and feet in the middle of a crowd until she was able to reach His hem (Luke 8:42–48 AKJV). It was then that she drew from Him and was healed in faith.

When we walk with God as a lifestyle of prayer and intimacy, we also walk with the same potential to God and all He has for us.

Chapter 20: Beauty without Limits

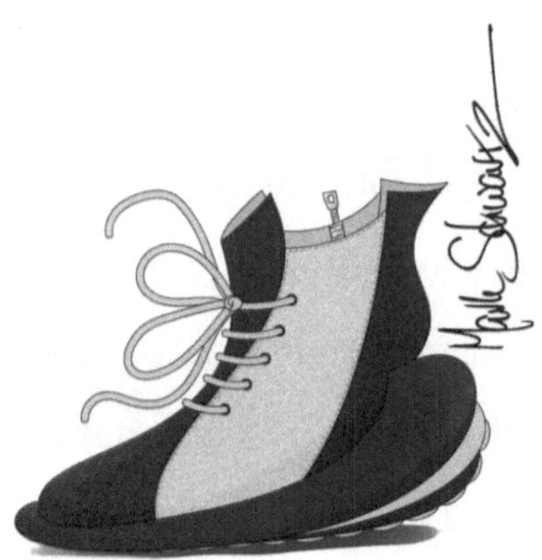

Beauty is not something you put on or wipe off. Beauty is a heart attitude authored by our everlasting God that you either accept or reject.
—Sandra J. Petrusaitis

Humor me for a while. Let's do a little experiment. Google the word "beauty" to see what results you get. Go ahead, I'll wait.

Pause here.

Chances are you'll get a page full of cosmetic and personal beauty websites. Okay, fine, it's the internet, not the book of life; however, the internet is often used to search the most popular categories. But I digress.

Who doesn't like a trip to the spa or the manicurist?

Right! But sometimes we tend to put beauty in categories or age brackets. We often associate beauty with youth and forget to appreciate the beauty that comes with time. I believe the real trap is believing that there is a limited definition of beauty.

We have a whole industry fertile with beauty options and treatments. Some women like makeup, while some women don't. But thank God that we have options.

Webster's definition of beauty says the word comes from the Middle English *beaute* and *bealte*, from the Anglo-French *bel* and *beau* (beautiful), and from the Latin *bellus* (pretty).

Furthermore, Webster defines beauty as "a beautiful person or thing; especially: a beautiful woman." What is wrong with this definition is the restriction of beauty to the realm of the visual. It's like saying just one facet of a sparkling diamond is beautiful.

If we only deemed those who are aesthetically appealing to be beautiful, then we would be limiting ourselves and others by failing to value all those other particulars that make us unique. If we used this definition as a measure of beauty, it would be like admiring one facet of a multifaceted, splendorous diamond when, in fact, it's the multiplicity of the diamond that makes it valuable and brilliant. It's the light bursting and bouncing from facet to facet that makes a diamond exquisitely beautiful. In the same way, you too were created to reflect beauty in the many facets and dimensions of your mind, body, and spirit. You have been created to sparkle and broadcast the one true light, the Father of heavenly lights Himself.

There are twelve definitions for beauty in Hebrew that give a richer, deeper meaning to the term.

Hadar means ornament, splendor, honor.

Hadarah means adornment, glory, holy adornment (of public worship), glory (of the king).

Howd means splendor, majesty, vigor.

Chamad means desire, covet, take pleasure in, delight in, desire, be desirable, delight greatly, desire greatly, desirableness, preciousness.

Yapheh means fair, beautiful, handsome.

Yophiy simply means beauty.

Na..em means be pleasant, be beautiful, be sweet, be delightful, be lovely.

No..am means kindness, pleasantness, delightfulness, beauty, favor, delightfulness, symbolic name of one of two staves, pleasantness.

Peh-ayr means headdress, ornament, turban.

Tseb-ee means beauty, glory, honor, beauty, decoration.

Tsuwr means rock, cliff.

Tiph'arah means beauty, splendor, glory of beauty, finery (of garments, jewels) glory of rank, renown as attribute of God, honor (or nation Israel) glorying, boasting (of individual).

Beauty on its own is in the eye of the beholder, as many

have said. However, true beauty in the way our God authored is meant to be seen, heard, tasted, and experienced so that His love, grace, and mercy can be experienced through the miracle of your life.

> *In that day the LORD of hosts will become a beautiful crown and a glorious diadem to the remnant of His people. (Isaiah 28:5 AKJV)*

Chapter 21: The Power of Repentance

A weapon of mass destruction.

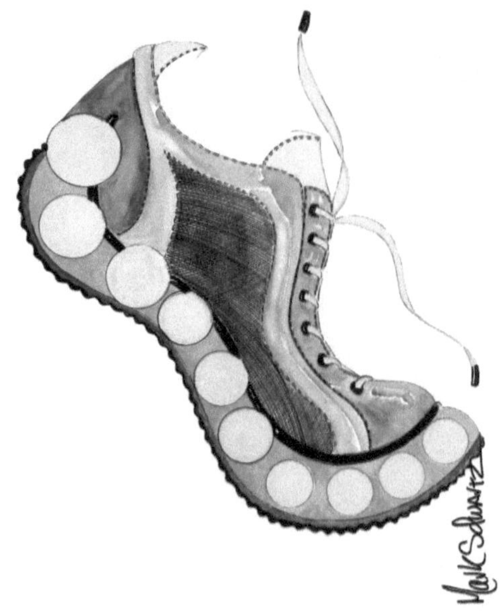

Repentance is a gift from heaven given to all who receive it through Jesus. Through this gift, we become sons and daughters of the Most High God (Ephesians 1:3-14 AKJV). Repentance is a power of unlimited, uncontainable, and indescribable force.

It is the living, pulsing, and ever-present power that brought Christ Jesus from death, hell, and the grave that you might live a miraculous life full of His glorious wonder.

Repentance in the Greek language is translated as "metamorphose" or "metamorphosis." In Matthew 3:2 (NKJV), we can read of that kind of repentance. It is a repentance intended to bring us to judge ourselves and our deeds before God and then choose to do it His way. It is a self-judgment that can happen only between you and Him. It's that place in your soul where only God and you really, really know the truth, your errors and deeds.

> *The will and the power we choose to change our mind and heart when we are wrong is what makes us truly human.*
> —*Sandra J. Petrusaitis*

The beauty of getting to that place in your soul where sin abides is that you can then be translated from sin into the kingdom of God, where all that is noble and wholesome and good abides. It's what God intended for you to abide in from the beginning of time. It's your identity, the one you yearn for and search for. And Christ, through His sacrifice by paying for our sins, is the way to get there.

Repentance is the bridge to reconciling with the Father. Christ is the only way to get there. It takes no pomp and circumstance to repent. This doesn't only happen in church. It's a deep and real experience; in a moment, you recognize that you are not right with Him. In that moment, His grace and compassion are waiting. For He is a loving and merciful Father. It is in that moment that He comes to cover your sin with His sacrifice. It's your place of vulnerability, when you are most weak, looking at your flaws.

Yet, your most powerful and protected moment is in Him. For when you are weak, He is strong. This posture of repentance is the place where walls are destroyed and any ground the enemy might have taken is regained. For no weapon formed against you will prosper. Repentance is a weapon of massive destruction in the kingdom of darkness. The enemy loses all footholds and cannot entangle or bind you. For greater is He who lives in you than he who is in the world (1 John 4:4 NKJV). Repent and rejoice! Rejoice!

References

Austin, P. (n.d.). https://www.preceptaustin.org/. Retrieved from
https://www.preceptaustin.org/

Biblegateway.com. (n.d.). Retrieved from http://www.
biblegateway.com

biblehub.com. (n.d.).

http://itakeoffthemask.com/words-of-wisdom/means-walk-god/.
(n.d.).

http://www.highheeledart.com/about-me/. (n.d.).

http://www.highheeledart.com/paintings/shoe-as-idea-collage-
50x45. (n.d.).

http://www.patheos.com/blogs/christiancrier/2015/07/27/top-7-
bible-verses-about-gods-direction/. (n.d.).

https://biblehub.com/psalms/68-6.htm. (n.d.).

https://everydayservant.com/top-19-bible-verses-walking-with-
god/. (n.d.).

https://www.kingjamesbibleonline.org/Bible-Verses-About-
Submission/. (n.d.).

https://www.kingjamesbibleonline.org/Bible-Verses-About-
Submission/. (n.d.).

https://www.openbible.info/topics/walking_with_god. (n.d.).

https://www.openbible.info/topics/walking_with_god.

https://www.thefreedictionary.com/storge. (2019, 01 25).

Retrieved from https://www.thefreedictionary.com/storge

www.ingramcontent.com/pod-product-compliance
Lightning Source LLC
Chambersburg PA
CBHW031128250726
48655CB00002B/563